SPINAL CORD INJURIES IN CHILDREN

SPINAL CORD INJURIES IN CHILDREN

by

JAMES E. WILBERGER, JR., M.D.

Clinical Assistant Professor of Neurosurgery,
University of Pittsburgh,
School of Medicine,
Pittsburgh, Pennsylvania
and
Associate Director,
Neurological Research,
Allegheny Singer Research Institute,
Allegheny General Hospital,
Pittsburgh, Pennsylvania

Futura Publishing Company, Inc.
Mount Kisco, New York
1986

Library of Congress Cataloging-in-Publication Data

Wilberger, James E.
  Spinal cord injuries in children.

  Includes bibliographies and index.
    1. Spinal cord—Wounds and injuries. 2. Children—
Wounds and injuries. I. Title. [DNLM: 1. Spinal
Cord Injuries—in infancy & childhood.
WL 400 W664s]
RD594.3.W53 1986   617′.482044   84-45919
ISBN 0-87993-264-3

Published by
Futura Publishing Company, Inc.
P.O. Box 330, 295 Main Street
Mount Kisco, New York 10549

L.C. No.: 85-45919
ISBN No.: 0-87993-264-3

CONTRIBUTORS

Parviz Baghai, MD, FACS
Clinical Assistant Professor,
Department of Neurosurgery,
University of Pittsburgh,
School of Medicine;
Department of Neurosurgery,
Allegheny General Hospital,
Pittsburgh, Pennsylvania

Anna J.L. Chorazy, MD, FAAP
Medical Director,
Rehabilitation Institute of Pittsburgh,
Pittsburgh, Pennsylvania

Sue Cooperman, MS, OTR/L
Director of Occupational Therapy,
Rehabilitation Institute of Pittsburgh,
Pittsburgh Pennsylvania

Ruth Ann Keen, LPT
Director of Physical Therapy,
Rehabilitation Institute,
Pittsburgh, Pennsylvania

Phyllis-Ann Mandella, RD
Director of Nutritional Services,
Rehabilitation Institute of Pittsburgh,
Pittsburgh, Pennsylvania

Mahnaz Tadjziechy, MD
Assistant Professor,
Department of Anesthesiology,
University of Pittsburgh,
School of Medicine,
Pittsburgh, Pennsylvania

Jan Titonis, MPH
Senior Program Coordinator,
Rehabilitation Institute of Pittsburgh,
Pittsburgh, Pennsylvania

Ann S. Valco, MD, FACC, FAAPMR
Pediatric Physiatrist,
Rehabilitation Institute of Pittsburgh,
Pittsburgh, Pennsylvania

Frank T. Vertosick Jr., MD
Department of Neurosurgery,
University of Pittsburgh,
School of Medicine,
Pittsburgh, Pennsylvania

PREFACE

Spinal cord injuries occur at the rate of approximately 7,000 to 8,000 per year in the United States.[11] While 50 percent of these injuries occur in individuals under 25 years of age, spinal injuries with major neurologic involvement are relatively uncommon in children and adolescents. It has been estimated that only 1 percent to 3 percent of all spinal injuries occur in individuals under 15 years of age (Fig. 1). When spinal injuries do occur in children and adolescents, anatomical and developmental factors predispose the upper cervical spine to the most severe injuries (in adults the most severe injuries occur in the lower cervical spine and thoracolumbar region). Because of this predisposition, children are more likely to suffer catastrophic neurologic loss, such as quadriplegia, from such injuries. Spinal cord injuries in children are more likely to occur in males than females by a ratio of 2 to 1, have a seasonal peak in the summer months, and are most often secondary to motor vehicle accidents, which account for one of every three spinal cord injuries in children.[5,6,9] The second most common cause is related to diving and other sport accidents (Fig. 2). The death rate of from 10 percent to 59 percent in children with serious spinal cord injuries emphasizes the seriousness of this problem.[1,2,4,7,8,10]

A serious spinal cord injury to a child can have devastating effects on the child and his family from not only a physical standpoint but from emotional and financial standpoints as well. In patients aged 0 to 14 years, 100 percent of paraplegics will survive up to 60 months, while 85 percent of quadriplegics will survive up to 60 months (Fig. 3). In 1985 dollars, the average acute hospital cost for a

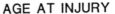

AGE AT INJURY

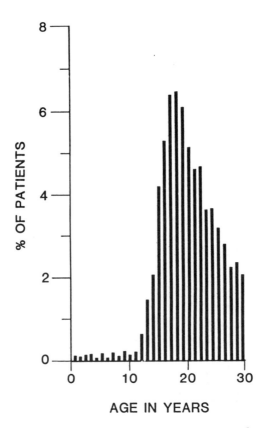

AGE IN YEARS

Figure 1. Age distribution of spinal cord injuries occurring in individuals up to age 30. Note that the majority of spinal cord injuries occur in the 18 to 25-year age range.

child with paraplegia was approximately $250,000. Acute hospital charges for a child with quadriplegia approached $300,000. Additionally, it has been estimated that the yearly annual expense of care for a child with quadriplegia or paraplegia approaches $50,000. Thus, the total annual cost of medical maintenance of children with severe spinal cord

Auto Accidents.......................71

Bicycle/Pedestrian Auto......14

Falls 78

Sports 21

Water Activities 19

Gunshot/Knife.......................7

Total....................210

Figure 2. Distribution of the causes of spinal cord injury in 210 children under 15 years of age.[1,3,8]

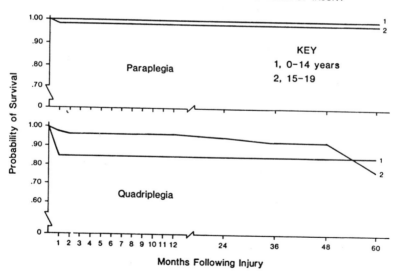

Figure 3. The long-term survival statistics of children with paraplegia and quadriplegia.

injuries approaches $75 to $125 million per year. As such maintenance may span the life of the individual, the total cost for each injury could exceed $1.5 million.[3,4,11]

Present therapy offers little hope for restitution of neurologic function, therefore, prevention of spinal cord injuries remains of paramount importance. Since motor vehicle accidents are the primary cause of spinal cord injuries in children, prevention lies in the development and implementation of effective child restraint systems. Many states are now in the process of passing legislation that would make safe child restraint systems mandatory in all vehicles. Hopefully, once this becomes a nationwide policy, the already small number of spinal cord injuries in children will drop by another 50 percent to 60 percent. Meanwhile, however, it remains of utmost importance for any physician involved in the acute care of the traumatized child to be able to recognize and acutely manage all aspects of spinal cord injury in the pediatric population.

Because spinal cord injuries in children and adolescents are not common, information relative to the diagnosis, immediate acute care, medical and surgical management of spinal fractures, and rehabilitation of the spinal cord injured child is fragmented and incomplete. This book will offer a comprehensive overview of the unique problems associated with spinal cord injury in children. The importance of being able to properly assess a young child with a suspected spinal cord injury, making the appropriate radiological diagnosis, and achieving immediate medical as well as spinal stabilization cannot be overemphasized. The guidelines presented in this book are intended to provide the information for state-of-the-art care for the spinal cord injured child.

REFERENCES

1. Anderson JM, Schutt AH: Spinal injury in children: A review of the 156 cases seen from 1950-1978. *Mayo Clin Proc* 55:499-504, 1980.
2. Babcock JL: Spinal injuries in children. *Pediatr Clin North Am* 22(2):487-500, 1975.

3. Bailey RW, Sherk HH (eds): *The Cervical Spine Research Society.* Philadelphia, J.B. Lippincott, 1983, pp 206-223.
4. Burke DC: Spinal cord trauma in children. *Paraplegia* 10:1-14, 1970.
5. Gaufin LM, Goodman SJ: Cervical spine injuries in infants. *J Neurosurg* 42:179-184, 1975.
6. Henrys P, Lyne ED, Lifton C, Salcicciotti G: Clinical review of cervical spine injuries in children. *Clin Orthop Relat Res* 129:172-176, 1977.
7. Hubbard DD: Injuries of the spine in children and adolescents. *Clin Orthop Relat Res* 100:56-66, 1974.
8. Kewalramani LS, Kraus JF, Sterling JM: Acute spinal cord lesions in the pediatric population: Epidemiological and clinical features. *Paraplegia* 18:206-219, 1980.
9. Ogden JA (ed): *Skeletal Injury in the Child.* Philadelphia, Lea & Febiger, 1982, pp 385-422.
10. Scher AT: Trauma of the spinal cord in children. *S Afr Med J* 42:2023-2025, 1976.
11. Young JS, Burns PE, Bowan AM, McCutchen R: *Spinal Cord Injury Statistics.* Phoenix, The Good Samaritan Medical Center, 1982, pp 11-15, 41-52.

ACKNOWLEDGMENTS

The author gratefully acknowledges the following individuals for their invaluable assistance in preparation of this book: Marge Zymanski, Doris Weyand, Diane Betrum, and Marsha McGee for their assistance with word processing; Keith Little and Valerie Hirsch of the Allegheny General Hospital Media Department for their assistance with illustrations; Theresa Westfall, RN, and Debbie Kubancek for their assistance with manuscript coordination.

CONTENTS

Chapter 1

ANATOMY AND BIOMECHANICS OF THE IMMATURE SPINE

Significant anatomical and biomechanical differences exist between the adult and pediatric spine. These differences account for the characteristic patterns of spinal injuries seen in children. Loose ligaments and joint capsules, in combination with the primarily cartilaginous nature of the infantile vertebrae contribute to characteristic x-ray patterns that must be understood when dealing with children with suspected spinal injuries. Some understanding of normal epiphyseal development, ongoing vertebral ossification, and the limits of physiological mobility in the pediatric spine is necessary for the proper assessment and treatment of children with spinal injuries.

EPIPHYSEAL DEVELOPMENT

Epiphyseal plates are ubiquitous in children. They are smooth, regular, and predictable in location. While a complete knowledge of the exact times of appearance and resolution of the epiphyseal plates in the spine is not necessary, some understanding of their typical appearance is important (Fig. 1).[1,2,4,5,6,30]

1

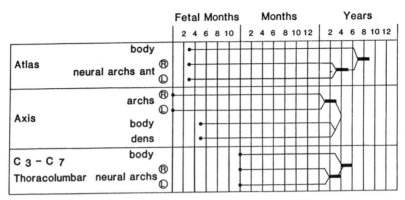

- Ossification Center Appears
- Synchondroses Fused

Figure 1. A chart outlining the appearance of ossification centers and the time to fusion of synchondroses in the immature spine. The majority of epiphyseal plates are fused by age six.

The Atlas

At birth, the atlas or C1 has three ossification centers—one for the body and one for each of the neural arches. The neural arches characteristically close by the third year of life to form a complete ring and subsequently fuse with the body of C1 by the seventh year (Fig. 2). These epiphyseal plates or synchondrosis can be readily seen, especially on open-mouth views of the atlas (Fig. 3). In the neonate the anterior arch of C1 will be discontinuous approximately 80 percent of the time.[1,6,19,30]

The Axis

The axis or C2 has four centers of ossification—one for each neural arch, one for the body of the C2, and one for the odontoid process (Fig. 4). The odontoid does not become completely fused with the body and neural arches of C2

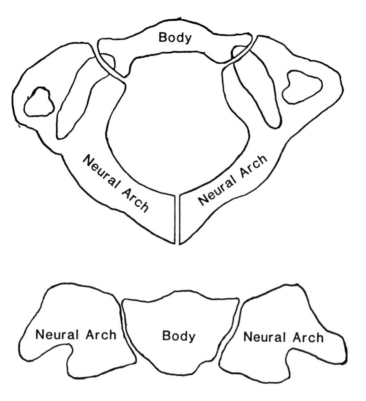

Figure 2. Schematic anatomical representation of ossification centers and epiphyseal plates of the atlas.

until approximately three to six years of age. The dens is separated from the body of the axis by a broad cartilaginous band, which in actuality corresponds to an intervertebral disc. This cartilaginous band gradually is ossified completely during early childhood.[1,6] This characteristic synchondrosis at the base of the dens is often mistaken for a fracture (Fig. 5). It can be seen in all children at three years of age and approximately 50 percent of children five years of age. Some authors have suggested that the odontoid synchondrosis may be seen as a thin line mimicking an undisplaced fracture up to age 11. Only rarely does this line persist into adult life.

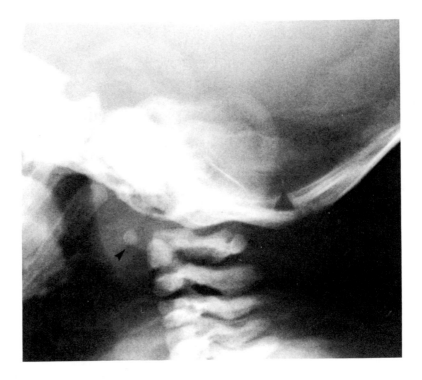

Figure 3. Incomplete ossification of the anterior arch of C1 (arrow) in a six-month-old child.

The tip of the odontoid is not ossified at birth. The cartilaginous odontoid tip is separated from the rest of the dens by a V-shaped cartilaginous plate. By three to six years of age ossification of the odontoid tip occurs and fusion with the body of the odontoid proceeds. Persistence of an unfused apical adontoid tip is known as an ossiculum terminale and has no pathologic significance.[14]

Os Odontoideum

Os odontoideum occurs when there is a complete separation of the odontoid from the body of the axis by a gap of

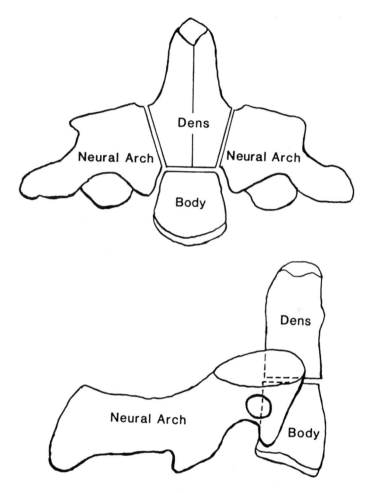

Figure 4. Schematic anatomical representation of ossification centers and epiphyseal plates of the axis.

varying widths. It was originally felt that this abnormality resulted from a failure of fusion of the odontoid with the axis.[10,11,13,32,34] However, recent information has suggested that the os odontoideum develops from a traumatic lesion resulting from an occult odontoid fracture occurring at an early age. Subsequent incomplete healing of the fracture

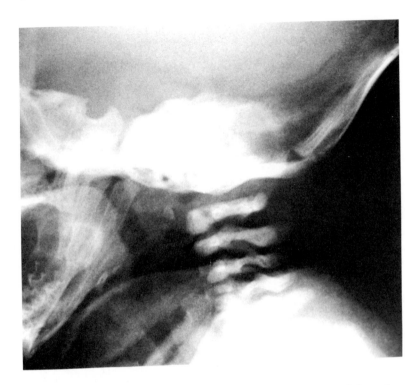

Figure 5A. *Characteristic synchondrosis at the base of the adontoid (arrow) in a six-month-old infant (A) and a seven-year-old child (B). This synchondrosis is present in up to 50 percent of children and should not be mistaken for a fracture.*

and bone resorption leads to an os odontoideum.[9,26] The importance of recognizing this congenital abnormality lies in the fact that clinically significant C1-2 subluxation with spinal cord compression can occur when an os odontoideum is present.

Lower Cervical, Thoracal Lumbar Spine

The C3 through C7, as well as all thoracic and lumbar vertebrae have a similar ossification pattern. Ossification

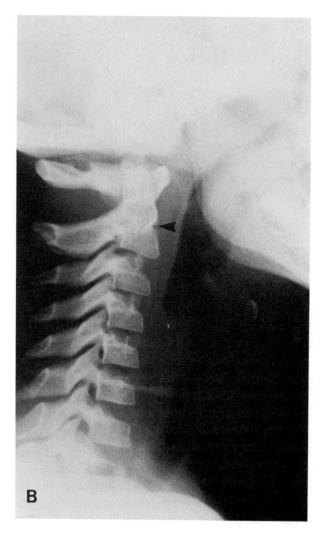

Figure 5B.

centers form in each of the two neural arches and in the vertebral body shortly after birth. Complete ossification with fusion of the neural arches to the vertebral body generally occurs by three to six years of age (Fig. 6). Complete

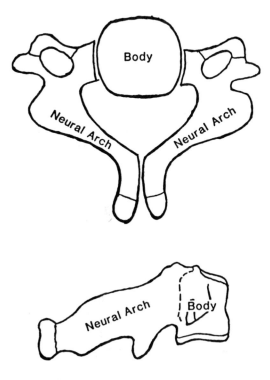

Figure 6. Schematic anatomical representation of the ossification centers and epiphyseal plates of a lower cervical vertebra.

fusion of the posterior neural arches generally occurs by two to three years of age and should not be confused with congenital anomalies such as spina bifida. On lateral x-rays the ossified vertebral bodies appear wedge-shaped and do not assume their characteristic rectangular shape until approximately seven years of age (Fig. 7).[6,8,21,25]

By eight years of age the cervical region as well as the thoracic and lumbar spine generally attain adult characteristics and epiphyseal lines no longer pose significant diagnostic problems.

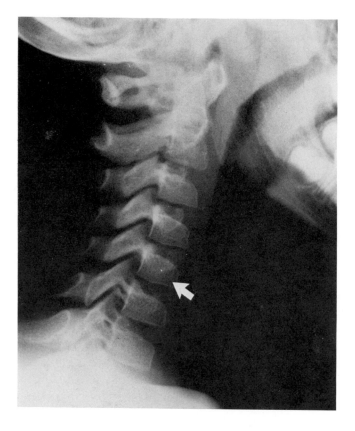

Figure 7. *Characteristic wedge-shaped cervical verte-bral bodies in a six-year-old. The wedging is particularly prominent at C5 (arrow).*

JOINT AND LIGAMENTOUS DEVELOPMENT

The geometry of the articulating surfaces of the joints and the elastic properties of the supporting ligaments are significantly different in the adult and pediatric spines. The elastic nature of these structures is much more pronounced in the child, making the pediatric spine a highly mobile structure. Knowledge of these differences is important in the diagnosis and management of pediatric spine pathology.

Characteristically the supporting ligaments help to maintain normal alignment by preventing excessive mobility in the vertebral bodies. The most important ligaments in this respect are the anterior and posterior longitudinal ligaments, which run the length of the spine. Additional supporting ligaments exist in the occipito-atlanto-axial region, which aid in preventing any excessive mobility in this area that could result in significant compromise of the lower brain stem or upper spinal cord.

The primary stability at the occipito-atlanto-axial articulation is provided by direct ligamentous attachments between the axis and the occiput. Because of the various motions it subserves, the atlas is only loosely connected to the occiput and axis by the weak, supporting occipitoatlantal membranes. The direct ligamentous attachments that provide stability of this joint are the tectorial membrane (continuation of the posterior longitudinal ligament), the lateral alar or check ligaments, the apical-dentate ligament, and the cruciate ligaments. The dens is tightly applied to the anterior arch of C1 by the thick transverse ligament (Fig. 8).[4,17,33]

In the pediatric spine, these ligaments have not achieved their normal elastic properties and, on occasion, will, with minor trauma, allow for abnormal mobility between the vertebral bodies. It has been suggested that the adult ligamentous characteristics are not attained until after age eight.[4]

The normal planes of the articulating surfaces of the facet joints also change significantly with growth. The facet joints provide vertebral body-to-vertebral body stability and allow for normal flexion and extension movement. In the lower cervical spine the facet joints have been noted to change from 55° to 70° in orientation, while in the upper cervical spine initial angles of as low as 30° have been re-

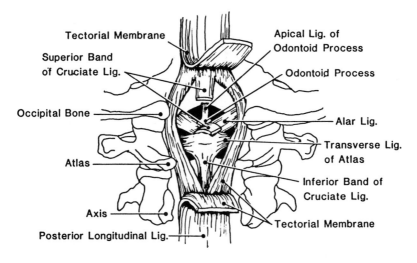

Figure 8. *The ligaments of the cranial vertebral junction.*

corded and gradually change to 60° to 70° by ten years of age. In addition to this change in orientation of the joints, the facets are not often well ossified until approximately seven to ten years of age and cannot exert any significant stability until complete ossification has been accomplished.[21,22]

BIOMECHANICS OF THE PEDIATRIC SPINE

The biomechanics of the spine are dependent on two primary factors (1) the geometry of the articulating joints or facets and (2) the mechanical properties of the ligaments. As noted previously, the immature spine has some specific developmental and anatomical factors that produce characteristic biomechanics and predispose it to certain fracture and spinal cord injury patterns when trauma is superimposed. The primary difference between adult and pediatric biomechanics is the increased physiological mobility of the pediatric spine, which is due to the following multiple factors: (a) ligamentous laxity, (b) incomplete ossification and shallow angulation of the facet joints, (c) incompletely ossified, wedge-shaped vertebral bodies, (d) underdeveloped neck musculature (Fig. 9).[12,15,18,23,24]

In children, motion in the lower cervical spine characteristically is different than in adults. With flexion and extension in adults, motion is greatest at the C5-6 level. In children, the greatest motion occurs at the C2-3 level and the fulcrum of motion gradually shifts downward as aging occurs. Adult spinal motion characteristics are usually developed by eight to ten years of age.[18,22] The joints of the upper cervical spine are complicated and will be dealt with separately.

As infantile vertebral bodies are primarily cartilagenous, overall lengthening of the immature spine readily occurs with axial loading. Axial loading with distraction of the spine can result in up to a two-inch elongation of the vertebral column. As a result, the spinal cord must also accommodate, otherwise irreversible injury would result. With flexion and extension, spinal cord segments individually can change by as much as 25 percent in order to prevent severe traction injury on the nervous tissue.[15,16,20]

Thus, the overall anatomical characteristics of the immature spine predispose it to excessive mobility. It is for this reason that children with significant spinal cord injuries may show no evidence of bony abnormalities on radiological investigation.

Atlanto-occipital Complex

The atlanto-occipital (A-O) complex is an extremely complicated articulation acting as a transition between the head and spine that provides mainly support and only limited motion.[11,17,30,33]

Flexion extension is the only significant movement allowed at the A-O articulation. The maximum degree of flex-

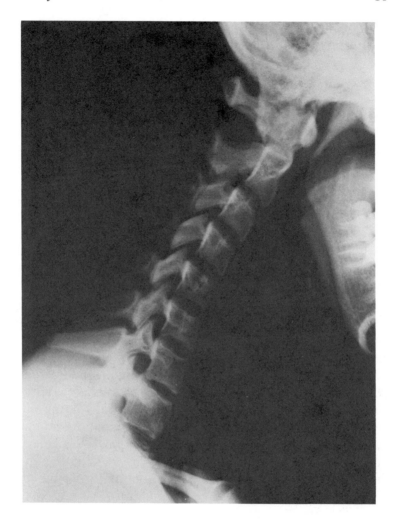

Figure 9. Characteristic flexion view of the cervical spine in a 10-year-old child. Notice that there is slight movement and angulation at the C2-3, C3-4, C4-5, and C5-6 levels. This is within normal physiological variation in a 10-year-old child due to ligamentous laxity and immature facet joints.

ion extension at this joint has been measured as approximately 13°. No rotation is allowed because of the shape of the occipital condyles and their articulation with the lateral masses of the atlas. A negligible amount of lateral bending (less than 12 percent) is allowed at the A-O articulation.

Atlantoaxial Articulations

The most important structure in the stability of the atlantoaxial joint is the dens.[11,19,33] The tip of the dens rests in a small articular facet in the back of the anterior arch of C1, while the transverse ligament closely binds the dens to the arch of C1. Paired accessory ligaments rise from the lateral masses of C2 and attach directly onto the dens slightly above the base. A pair of alar ligaments run inferiolaterally from the occipital condyles to the superolateral aspects of the dens to form a firm attachment. An unpaired apical ligament runs from the ventral aspect of the foramen magnum and inserts centrally at the tip of the dens (Fig. 8). All of these ligamentous attachments allow for an extremely stable joint at the same time allowing flexion and extension, rotation, vertical approximation, and lateral gliding at the C1-2 level. Approximately 10 percent of flexion extension occurs at the C1-2 level. Bony contact between the rim of the foramen magnum and the odontoid tip prevents excessive forward flexion at this level thus protecting the upper cervical cord and brain stem. Likewise, significant hyperextension is prevented by the contact of the posterior arch of C1 with the occiput and the tectorial membrane. Greater than 50 percent rotation is allowed at the C1-2 articulation because of the horizontal orientation of the articular surfaces between the atlas and the axis. When rotation occurs at this level, the odontoid process serves as a pivot point. Rotation is controlled to some extent by the alar ligaments. However, extreme degrees of rotation are not without potential complications. The vertebral arteries, having entered the foramina transversaria at C6, run over the articular surface of C1-2 before entering the foramen magnum. With only 30° of rotation, a significant kinking of the contralateral vertebral artery has been noted. The degree of kinking increases with increasing rotation. By 45° of rotation, the ipsilateral vertebral artery also begins to kink. If blood flow in both arteries is compromised or if one artery is maldeveloped, brain stem ischemia may occur. Thus, the possibility of significant vascular injury occurring in conjunction with spinal injuries must always be borne in mind.

C2-3 Pseudosubluxation

The entity of C2-3 pseudosubluxation provides a good example of the excessive mobility of the pediatric spine as related to ligamentous laxity and facet joint orientation.[3,7,15]

In otherwise normal children, a shift of the axis in relation to C3 may be seen on lateral x-ray views in forward flexion and hyperextension. Characteristically the axis slides forward and tilts downward (Fig. 10). This pseudosubluxation at C2-3 may be seen in up to 40 percent of children under eight years of age with more than 50 percent of these children having a 3 mm or greater degree of shift. This hypermobility of the C2-3 segment has been well studied and is directly related to ligamentous and joint capsule laxity as well as the immature development and horizontal orientation of the younger vertebral facet joints.[25] Over the age of ten, C2-3 pseudosubluxation is not seen because of the subsequent development of the ligaments and the orientation of the facet joints. True C2-3 subluxation can be differentiated from pseudosubluxation by forced hyperextension—in the child with true C2-3 subluxation the forward shift of the axis on the C3 cannot be reduced whereas in pseudosubluxation, the shift is always reduced by extension.[28,29,31]

The importance of C2-3 pseudosubluxation is in em-

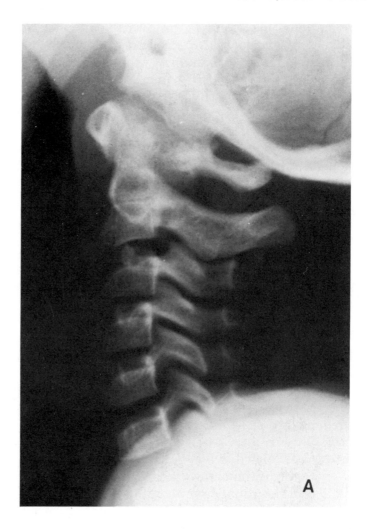

Figure 10A. C2–3 pseudosubluxation in a 7-year-old girl. Minimal malalignment is noted at the C2-3 level on neutral films (A). The C2-3 subluxation is accentuated on flexion (B) but reduced on extension (C).

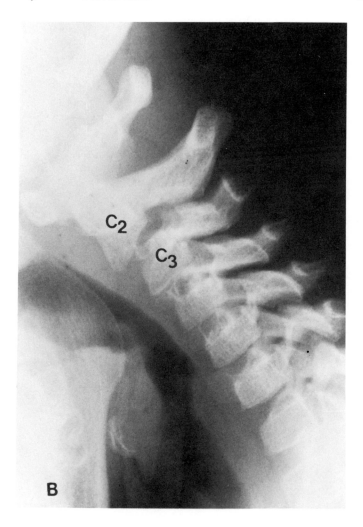

Figure 10B.

phasizing that this is a normal variant requiring no specific treatment or further diagnostic intervention. A similar pseudosubluxation can sometimes be seen at the C3-4 level and occurs in approximately 15 percent of children under age ten.

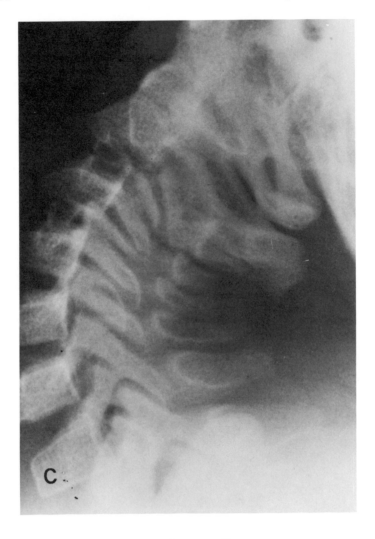

Figure 10C.

REFERENCES

1. Bailey DK: The normal cervical spine in infants and children. *Radiology* 59:712, 1952.
2. Bailey DK: The normal cervical spine in infants and children. *Radiology* 59:712–719, 1952.
3. Bailey RW, Sherk HH (eds): *The Cervical Spine Research Society*. Philadelphia, J.B. Lippincott, 1983, pp 206–223.
4. Bardeen CR: The development of the skeleton and of the connective tissues, in Keibel F, Maul FP (eds): *Manual of Human Embryology*. Philadelphia, J.B. Lippincott, 1910, pp 398–427.
5. Camp JD, Gilley EJL: Diagramatic chart showing time of appearance of the various centers of ossification and period of union. *Am J Roentgenol* 26:905, 1931.
6. Carpenter EB: Normal and abnormal growth of the spine. *Clin Orthop* 2:49, 1961.
7. Cattell HS, Filtzer DL: Pseudo-subluxation and other normal variations in the cervical spine in children. *J Bone Jt Surg* 47A(7):1295–1309, 1965.
8. Ehrenhaft JL: Development of the vertebral column as related to certain congenital and pathological changes. *Surg, Gynecol, Obstet* 76:282–292, March, 1943.
9. Fielding JW, Griffin PP: Os odondoiteum—an acquired lesion. *J Bone Jt Surg* 56A:187–190, 1974.
10. Fielding JW, Hessinger RN, Hawkins RJ: Os odontoideum. *J Bone Jt Surg* 62A(3):376–383, 1980.
11. Garber JN: Abnormalities of the atlas and the axis vertebrae—congenital and traumatic. *J Bone Jt Surg* 49A:1792, 1974.
12. Glasauer FE, Cares HL: Biomechanical features of traumatic paraplegia in infancy. *The J of Trauma* 13(II):166–170, 1973.
13. Hensinger RN, Fielding JW, Hawkins RJ: Congenital anomalies of the odontoid process. *Orthop Clin North America* 9:901–925, 1978.
14. Hensinger RN, Fielding JW, Hawkins RJ: Congenital anomalies of the odontoid process. *Orthop Clin North America* 9:909–912, 1978.
15. Hohl M: Normal motions in the upper portion of the cervical spine. *J Bone Jt Surg* 44A(8):1777–1779, 1964.
16. Hohl M, Hills B: Normal motions in the upper portion of the cervical spine. *J Bone Jt Surg* 46A(8):1777–1779, 1964.
17. Hohl M, Baker HR: The atlantoaxial joint. *J Bone Jt Surg* 46A:17–39, 1954.
18. Johnson RM: Some new observations on the functional anatomy of the lower cervical spine. *Clin Orthop* 111:192, 1975.
19. Naik DR: Cervical spinal canal in normal infants. *Clin Radiol* 21:323, 1970.
20. O'Brien MS (ed): *Pediatric Neurological Surgery*. New York, Raven Press, 1978, pp 306–312.
21. Ogdan JA: *Skeletal Injury in the Child*. Philadelphia, Lea & Febiger, 1982, pp 385–422.

22. Penning L: Normal movement of the cervical spine. *Am J Roentgenol* 130:317–326, 1978.
23. Penning L: Normal movement of the spine. *Am J Roentgeno* 130:317, 1978.
24. Roaf R: Vertebral growth and its mechanical control. *J Bone Jt Surg* 42B:40, 1960.
25. Sherk HH, Schut L, Lane JM: Fractures and dislocations of the cervical spine in children: Pseudo-subluxations and other variations. *Orthop Clin North America* 7(3):593–604, 1976.
26. Stillwell WT, Fielding JW: Acquired os odontoideum. *Clin Orthop* 135:71, 1978.
27. Sullivan CR, Brower AJ, Harris LE: Hypermobility of the cervical spine in children: A pitfall in the diagnosis of cervical dislocation. *Am J Surg* 93:636–640, 1958.
28. Sullivan CR, Brower AJ, Harris LE: Hypermobility of the cervical spine in children: Pitfall in the diagnosis of cervical dislocation. *Am J Surg* 9:636–639, 1948.
29. Swischuk LE: Anterior displacement of C2 in children: Physiological or Pathologic? *Pediatr Radiol* 122:759–763, 1977.
30. Torklus DV, Gehle W: *The Upper Cervical Spine*. New York, Grune & Stratton, pp 10–95, 1972.
31. Townsend EH, Rowe ML: Mobility of the upper cervical spine in health and disease. *Pediatrics* 10:567–574, 1952.
32. Truex RC, Johnson CH: Congenital anomalies of the upper cervical spine. *Orthop Clin North America* 9(4):891–900, 1978.
33. White AA, Panjebi M: The clinical biomechanics of the occipital-atlanto-axial complex. *Orthop Clin North America* 9(4):867–878, 1978.
34. Wollin D: The os odontoideum. *J Bone Jt Surg* 45A:1459, 1963.

Chapter 2

RADIOLOGICAL EVALUATION OF SPINAL TRAUMA

The injured child's spine can readily become a radiological diagnostic enigma. Multiple epiphyseal plates, the unique architecture of the immature vertebral bodies, incomplete vertebral ossification, and the characteristic hypermobility due to ligamentous laxity make radiological evaluation of the immature spine hazardous. Since fractures and dislocations of the spine are uncommon in the child, one must constantly bear in mind the normal radiology of the pediatric spine, which must be differentiated from traumatically induced abnormalities. To further complicate matters in the radiological evaluation, the entity of spinal cord injury without radiographic abnormality, which occurs in up to 20 percent of children under 15 years of age and which can result in severe spinal cord injury without observable radiographic abnormality, must constantly be considered when dealing with severely injured children.

The initial diagnostic evaluation should always include plain radiographs of the cervical and/or thoracolumbar spine. Additional useful information can often be obtained by performing flexion and extension views particularly when dealing with cervical spine abnormalities, however, extreme caution must be taken if instability is strongly suspected. To better interpret plain radiographs or to better delineate a definite abnormality, conventional biplane tomography or computerized axial tomography often prove extremely helpful. Likewise, myelography is sometimes necessary in the complete evaluation of the spinal cord injury. Currently, information is being accumulated concerning the usefulness of magnetic resonance imaging in spinal trauma. It is extremely important to understand the indications for proceeding with further radiological investigations when confronted with an abnormal plain spine film in an injured child. It is also important to understand that, because of the dynamic nature of the growth and development of the pediatric spine, serial radiographic examination may be necessary to diagnose injuries or progressive spinal deformities.

NORMAL PEDIATRIC SPINE RADIOGRAPHS

As in the evaluation of adult cervical spinal injuries, the first principle in evaluating the pediatric cervical spine is to clearly visualize all seven cervical vertebrae. Constructing four lines on the lateral view can be helpful in assessing the vertebral alignment and detecting any spinal canal impingement (Fig. 1). A smooth gentle curve, convex anteriorly should be formed by a line drawn down the anterior border of the vertebral bodies (Fig. 1, line a). Similar curves should be formed when lines are drawn down the posterior border of the vertebral bodies (Fig. 1, line b), the anterior margins of the bases of the spinous processes (Fig. 1, line c), and the tips of the spinous processes. The alignment of the facet joints and the relationships of the spinous processes are best seen on anteroposterior views (Fig. 2).

The most frequent error in evaluating suspected cervical spinal injury is failure to obtain clear visualization of the C7-T1 level. This usually poses little problem in children, however, occasionally a swimmer's view is necessary to adequately visualize this region. If the C7-T1 level cannot be visualized by conventional methods, the neck should be

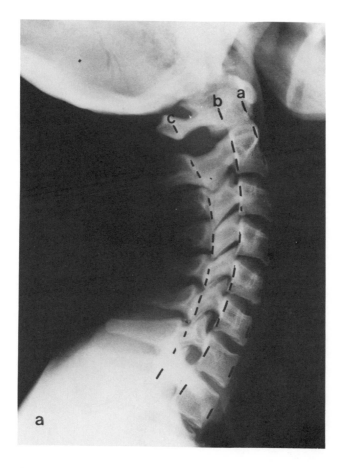

Figure 1A. Normal lateral cervical spinal films in an adolescent (a), a 7-year-old (b), and an infant (c). The dotted lines as outlined on Figure A refer to the normal anatomical alignment, which should be checked in all spine films.

stabilized with a collar or sandbags and tomography performed. The alignment of the vertebral bodies and the facet joints should be carefully evaluated in the AP and lateral radiographs. Any malalignment should be investigated further. Any bony abnormalities also should be studied carefully and investigated further.

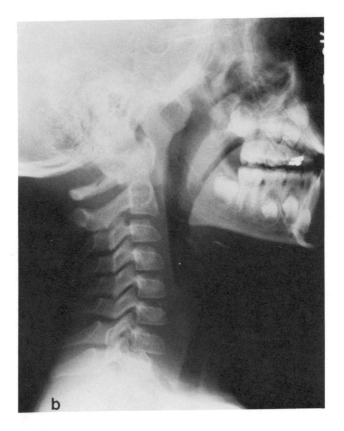

Figure 1B.

Occasionally, subtle bony injuries to the cervical spine may result in significant soft tissue swelling. In the child, the retropharyngeal soft tissue is most often affected. The space between the anterior edge of the upper cervical vertebrae and the air column of the pharynx should be a maximum of two-thirds thickness of the second cervical vertebra. Below the C3-4 level, the prevertebral soft tissue should not exceed the width of the vertebral body. On occasion, a prevertebral radiolucent fat stripe may be visualized. The position of this fat stripe should be closely opposed to

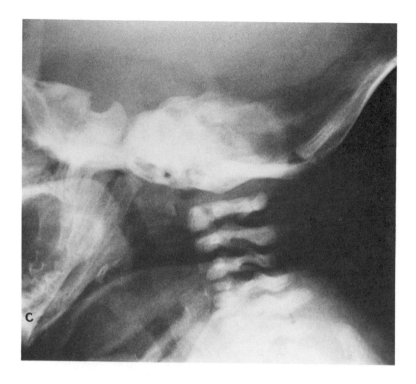

Figure 1C.

the anterior margin of the vertebral body. Abnormally wide prevertebral fat tissue spaces or displacement of the fat stripe in the absence of obvious bony abnormalities should lead to more detailed investigation.

When evaluating the C1-C2 region, careful attention must be given to the distance separating the anterior arch of C1 and the odontoid process. In the adult, the C1-dens distance is normally less than 2 mm. However, in the child, the anterior arch of C1 and the dens may be normally separated by as much as 5 mm because of the laxity of the transverse dental ligament in the child (Fig. 3). If any question exists about the pathologic nature of the C1-dens distance, flexion extension views are often helpful in clarifying this question.

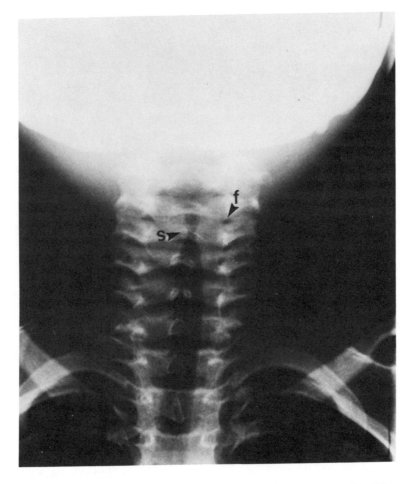

Figure 2. Normal AP cervical spine film in a 7-year-old. The spinous processes are all aligned (s) and facet joints (f) are symmetrical.

Under normal circumstances no change in the C1-dens distance should occur. The lucent line at the base of the dens (subdental synchondrosis) may persist up to 11 years of age and should not be mistaken for a fracture. Pseudosubluxation of up to 3 to 4 mm of C2 on C3 occurs in up to 40

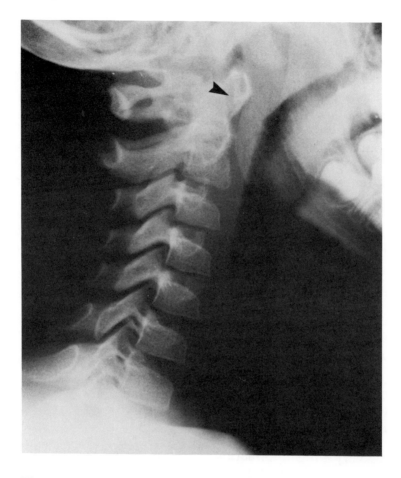

Figure 3. Normal lateral cervical spine film in an 11-year-old. Note the C1-dens distance of approximately 4 mm (arrow).

percent of normal children below eight years of age. A similar abnormality can be seen at the C3-4 level in up to 20 percent. If there is any question about the pathologic nature of subluxation at C2-3 or C3-4, then flexion-extension views would be helpful. A true subluxation will not reduce with flexion and extension.

Immature vertebral bodies are wedged anteriorly and do not assume their normal adult configuration until after ten years of age. This anterior wedging should not be mistaken for compression fractures. Additionally, the immature spinous process often has a secondary ossification center that should not be confused with an avulsion fracture.

Similarly, in the thoracolumbar spine, the normal anterior wedging of the vertebral bodies should not be mistaken for pathologic fractures. Additionally, lateral thoracic or lumbar spine films may show a vertically oriented cleft that represents a large nutrient vessel canal and should not be considered abnormal. Since osseous union of the posterior aspect of the neural arches in the thoracolumbar spine does not occur until two to four years of age, this lack of fusion should not be interpreted as a fracture in children in this age range.

By ten years of age, the pediatric spine has attained adult characteristics, both anatomically and radiographically, and the radiographs of the spine should be interpreted based on adult criteria.

ATLAS FRACTURES

Very little information exists as to the occurrence of atlas fractures in children.[11,18] The usual mechanism for fractures of the atlas involves axial compression of the head with downward displacement of the occipital condyles into the lateral masses of C1. This exerts a chisellike effect that may cause a bursting fracture of the ring of C1 (Jefferson's fracture). The bursting usually occurs in four places—two anteriorly and two posteriorly (Fig. 4). If the axial compressive force is eccentrically applied, occasionally single or multiple fractures may occur through the ring of C1 anteriorly or posteriorly or through the lateral masses of C1 (Fig. 5). This injury is rare in children—there have been

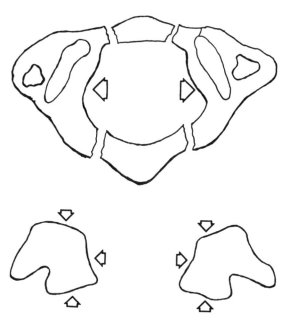

Figure 4. A direct blow to the vertex of the head produces a chisellike effect on C1 resulting in a burst or Jefferson's fracture. This schematic representation of an atlas fracture demonstrates the forces involved resulting in bony disruption (arrows).

only two cases reported in the literature. The flexibility of the cartilaginous synchondrosis in the ring of C1 is the most likely reason that this type of fracture is rare in children.[10]

If the transverse dental ligament remains intact when a Jefferson's fracture occurs, the plain lateral radiograph will be normal, unless retropharyngeal soft tissue swelling develops. If the ligament is disrupted, the C1-dens distance will be abnormally wide. The open-mouth odontoid view is important in evaluation for the presence of this type of fracture. Normally, the lateral margins of the articular facets of C1 will align with the lateral margins of the lateral masses

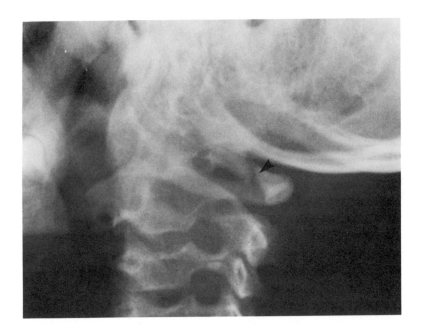

Figure 5. A single fracture through the posterior ring of C1 in a 6-year-old child resulting from eccentric compression of the atlas.

of C2. If the ring of C1 is fractured, the lateral masses of C1 will be displaced laterally relative to those of C2. If only one C1 ring fracture is present then only one lateral mass will be displaced. Care must be taken not to mistake the normal C1-C2 alignment that occurs secondary to rotation at this joint with the malalignment secondary to C1 fracture (Fig. 6).

   If such a fracture is suspected based on the clinical evaluation of the mechanism of injury or on plain radiographic abnormalities, then a computerized axial tomographic scan is excellent in visualizing the extent of atlas fractures.

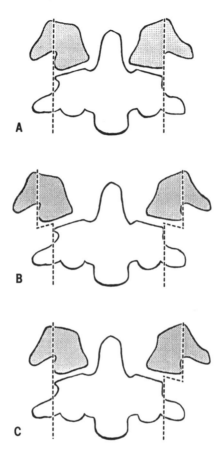

Figure 6. The normal C1-2 alignment is represented by the schematic drawing (A). A typical Jefferson's fracture with bilateral, lateral mass displacement is shown in (B). However, rotation at the C1-2 level produces an apparent lateral displacement of one lateral mass and should not be mistaken for a C1 fracture (C).

ATLANTOAXIAL SUBLUXATION

Isolated atlantoaxial subluxation occurs secondary to rupture of the transverse dental ligament as well as disruption of the supportive ligaments of the C1-2 articulation (alar ligaments, cruciate ligaments, apical ligament). C1-2 subluxation occasionally is due to trauma but is more commonly associated with inflammatory processes such as pharyngitis, tonsillitis, and juvenile rheumatoid arthritis. Nontraumatic C1-2 subluxation is known as Griesel's syndrome.[15,16,19]

Traumatic transverse ligament rupture is rare in children. The transverse ligament is stronger than the odontoid process because the dens is incompletely ossified and has a cartilaginous basal synchondrosis. Thus, the dens will fracture before the ligament ruptures, secondarily resulting in C1-2 subluxation. However, if the transverse ligament is weakened by an inflammatory process it may be predisposed to rupture. Traumatic subluxation of C1 on C2 occurs as a result of a severe flexion injury.

When C1-2 subluxation does occur, the atlas slides anteriorly resulting in an increased distance between the anterior arch of C1 and the dens (Fig. 7). In children, this distance should be considered abnormal if it exceeds 5 mm.

If questions arise concerning C1-2 subluxation based on plain radiographs, flexion-extension views are often helpful in delineating the exact nature of the abnormality. With flexion-extension views, the C1-dens interval should remain constant.

Another diagnostic x-ray sign of C1-2 subluxation is forward displacement of the posterior arch of the atlas. This can be recognized as a "step-off" in the normally smooth line made by the bases of the spinous processes (Fig. 1, line c).

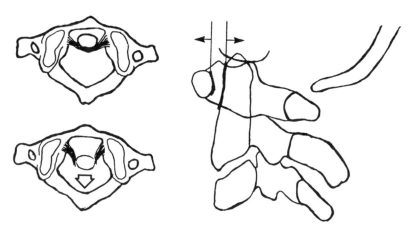

Figure 7. Schematic representation of C1-2 subluxation. The increased C-1 arch-dens distance is secondary to rupture of the transverse ligament and posterior displacement of the dens.

ATLANTO-OCCIPITAL DISLOCATION

Atlanto-occipital (A-O) dislocation is an extremely rare and dangerous injury. Only 14 cases have been reported in the literature, and of these, only eight patients have survived. However, the actual incidence of true atlanto-occipital dislocation may not be recognized because such an injury may result in cervicomedullary compression with instantaneous death.[14]

Because of the degree of motion allowed at the atlanto-occipital articulation, the atlas is only loosely connected to the occiput by a series of occipitoatlantal membranes. In adults, steep inclination of the atlanto-occipital joint provides considerable stability. However, in children, because of the shallow articular surfaces of the atlas and the small size of the occipital condyles, stability in this area is almost entirely dependent on ligamentous integrity. Additionally, congenital defects at the base of the skull may predispose the child to this type of injury. With ligamentous rupture, forward slippage of the occiput on C1 is possible, which may result in significant lower brain stem compression.[6]

The radiological diagnosis of atlanto-occipital dislocation can be extremely difficult. The mechanism of injury is characteristically a severe deceleration force, such as occurs in head-on collisions. Thus, radiographic recognition of this injury depends on identification of the malalignment of the odontoid with respect to the anterior edge of the foramen magnum (basion) and the malalignment of the posterior arch of the atlas with respect to the posterior edge of the foramen magnum (opisthion). Three sets of radiographic criteria have been advocated in making the diagnosis.

1. The dens-basion distance (DB) (Fig. 8, line a).
2. The distance between the posterior edge of the mandible and the anterior arch of C1 compared to the distance between the posterior edge of the mandible and the dens (Fig. 8, lines b,c).
3. The BC/OA ratio; BC (line e, Fig. 8) representing the distance between the basion (B) and the posterior arch of the C1 and O-A (line d, Fig. 8) representing the distance between the opisthion and the anterior arch of C1.

Specific numeric criteria have been carefully established for all three methods of diagnosing A-O dislocation. However, the third method, the BC/OA ratio is generally preferred because it is totally unaffected by the rotation, flexion, or extension.[14]

With careful measurement, the BC/OA ratio should always be less than 1.0, if normal C1 occipital anatomical alignment is present. If the ratio is greater than 1, then there has been some slippage of the occiput relative to C1, strongly suggestive of an atlanto-occipital dislocation.

If the radiographic criteria cannot be definitively established on plain radiographs and suspicion of A-O dislocation is high on a clinical basis, then biplane tomography of

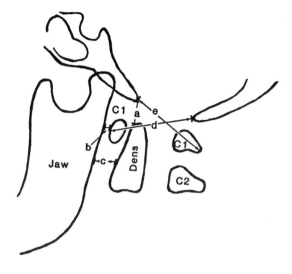

Figure 8. Schematic representation of the methods of making the radiological diagnosis of atlanto-occipital dislocation. (a) dens-basion distance; (b) distance from the posterior edge of the mandible to the anterior arch of C1; (c) distance from the posterior edge of the mandible to the dens; (d) distance from the opisthion to the anterior arch of C1; (e) distance between the basion and the posterior arch of C1.

the occipital C1 region may be helpful in demonstrating displacement of the dens laterally relative to the midpoint between the occipital condyles. Computerized tomographic scanning may also be helpful and delineate any possible associated fractures.

AXIS FRACTURES

Fractures of the Dens

Fractures of the dens are relatively rare in children under seven years of age and are extremely rare in children under three years of age. There are less than ten reported cases occurring in children under the age of three. The diagnosis of a dens fracture on a radiological basis can often be confusing when there is a coexisting ossiculum terminale, os odontoideum, or congenital absence of the dens. However, it is felt by many authors that the os odontoideum and congenital absence of the dens occur secondary to unrecognized trauma with associated fracture, subsequent nonhealing, and eventual bone resorption. For this reason, it is extremely important to recognize a dens fracture when it does occur.[8,17]

In most cases, fractures of the dens are associated with major trauma and are not difficult to diagnose on a radiographic basis. However, in some cases, the only clue to a fracture of the dens may be some retropharyngeal soft tissue swelling.

Dens fractures can occur secondary to either forced hyperextension or hyperflexion of the head. With hyperflexion injuries and associated transverse ligament rupture, the dens is displaced anteriorly with secondary forward subluxation of C1 on C2. With hyperextension, the dens is displaced posteriorly with associated posterior subluxation of C1 on C2. If the transverse ligament does not rupture, alignment between C1 and C2 generally remains normal.

Dens fractures tend to occur at different levels in the C2 vertebra in adults and children. On lateral plain radiographs of the adult, the fracture line through the dens generally occurs slightly above the level of the superior articulating facets of C1 and C2. In children, the fracture is usually well below the level of the facets and into the body of the C2. Characteristically, when a fracture line occurs through the base of the dens in children, it obliterates the normal epiphyseal growth plate that is usually present (dental synchondrosis). For this reason, it is felt that dens fractures in children are epiphyseal separations or slips rather than true bony fractures. Recognition of this fact has important therapeutic implications.

Plain lateral films are usually sufficient to make the diagnosis of dens fracture. In children who have sustained significant injuries and who are in considerable pain, it is often difficult and usually unnecessary to obtain open-mouth views of the odontoid process. If the plain films are not diagnostic and suspicion is high for a fracture of the dens, then the diagnosis can be confirmed by plain tomography or computerized tomographic scanning.[2]

HANGMAN'S FRACTURE

Hangman's fractures also are quite rare in children. There have been only two reported cases occurring in children under three years of age. A hangman's fracture consists of bilateral C2 pedicle fractures with associated subluxation of the body of C2 on C3.

The mechanism of injury is generally acute hyperextension. The hangman's fracture results from displacement of the C2 vertebral body upward and the inferior articular facets of C2 downward—resulting in bilateral C2 pedicle fractures. With both pedicles fractured, there is no bony support to prevent the body of C2 from slipping forward on C3. Because of the anatomical relationship between the dens and C1, with this injury the axis subluxes anteriorly as well. Occasionally, because of associated neck muscle spasm, the spine may be held rigidly fixed and the subluxation not appreciated.

Hangman's fractures are usually evident on plain lateral radiographs. However, if a fracture of this level is suspected but not readily identifiable, it is important to obtain films in a mild degree of flexion, which will always bring out the subluxation and help in identification of the fracture line. If plain films are not helpful, then biplane tomography or CT scan is generally useful in establishing the diagnosis.[20]

ATLANTOAXIAL ROTARY SUBLUXATION

Rotary subluxation of the atlas on the axis is a relatively common problem that occurs as a result of unrecognized or minor trauma and typically presents in the child with painful torticollis or restricted, painful neck motion. Rotary subluxation occurs when the atlas locks in rotation on the axis. This is characteristically a unilateral phenomenon involving the lower facet of C1 rotated forward on the corresponding facet of C2. The mechanism of this rotary injury is unknown, but may be associated with interposition of the capsular ligaments between the atlas and the axis, some irregularity in the facet joints secondary to an occult fracture, or to complete dislocation of the facet joints between C1 and C2.[3,4]

Open-mouth views on plain radiographs of the upper cervical spine are necessary to establish the diagnosis. The odontoid is characteristically asymmetrically placed between the lateral articular masses of the atlas on the open-mouth view. The lateral mass of the atlas that is rotated forward on C2 will appear wider and closer to the midline than the opposite lateral mass which appears narrower and farther away from the midline. Additionally, on the side where the atlas is rotated backward on C2, the joint space between the lateral masses of C1 and C2 will be obscured because of apparent overlapping (Fig. 9). If this phenomenon is observed, it is essential to rule out the possibility that the asymmetrical placement of the dens and abnormal lateral mass appearances are secondary to involuntary rotation of the head. Therefore, it is necessary to obtain films with the head rotated 10° to 15° to both the right and left sides. In true rotary subluxation, the asymmetrical placement of the odontoid relative to the articular masses of the atlas will remain unchanged. An additional aid in the radiological diagnosis of rotary subluxation is the location of the spinous process of C2. With voluntary rotation, the spine of C2 moves in a direction opposite to the chin. In true rotary subluxation, the tip of the spine of C2 will remain on the same side as the chin because C1 and C2 are locked and moving as a single unit.[4]

Should questions remain about the possibility of rotary subluxation being present, biplane tomography may be helpful. Tomograms should demonstrate that the lateral masses of the atlas are in different coronal planes secondary to the rotation and may erroneously suggest that one lateral mass is absent. Another extremely useful test is CT scanning, which will always demonstrate the pathology involved with rotary subluxation. Unilateral joint subluxation

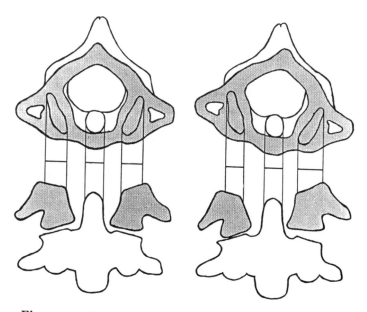

Figure 9. Diagram of assymetric placement of the odontoid and forward rotation of one lateral mass of C1 that is characteristic of atlantoaxial rotary subluxation.

with associated facet locking can be clearly seen on axial CT cuts.

C2-3 SUBLUXATION

In spite of the characteristic hypermobility of the upper cervical spine in children and the common occurrence of C2-3 pseudosubluxation, traumatic C2-3 subluxation rarely occurs. C2-3 subluxation occurs as a result of acute flexion injury to the upper cervical spine. As opposed to pseudosubluxation, the degree of displacement of C2 anteriorly on C3 is generally greater than 4 mm in traumatic subluxation. An extremely important differentiating point of true subluxation from pseudosubluxation is that in traumatic subluxation, the anterior displacement of C2 on C3 is present not only in the neutral position but persists in flexion and extension. Therefore, it is extremely important in a child in whom a C2-3 subluxation is suspected to obtain flexion-extension views. Tomography is usually not helpful unless there are associated posterior element fractures.[11,12]

The possibility of C2-3 subluxation emphasizes the importance of considering serial radiographs in children with suspected spinal injuries. In C2-3 pseudosubluxation, serial radiographs in the neutral position and in flexion and extension will show no significant change in the degree of subluxation. However, if a true traumatic C2-3 subluxation has occurred, then serial radiographs may show progressive deformity with further anterior displacement of C2 on C3.[18]

The entity of C2-3 subluxation raises the importance of considering the clinical examination to guide the radiological investigation in spinal trauma. A child who has suffered an acute flexion injury with local tenderness and neck spasm deserves extremely careful radiological evaluation to rule out the possibility of associated spinal injury.

FRACTURES AND DISLOCATIONS
OF THE LOWER CERVICAL SPINE

Fractures and dislocations of the cervical spine below the level of C3 are not common in children. In adults, 85 percent of fractures and dislocations in the cervical region occur below the level of C3, in children only 30 percent occur below this level. Locked facets, either unilateral or bilateral, which are so common in adults with lower cervical spinal injuries, are not seen in children.[7]

The most common fractures of the lower cervical spine in children are wedge-compression fractures. The mechanisms of these injuries are characteristically flexion associated with axial loading. When compression fractures occur, there is usually associated disruption of the posterior longitudinal ligament that allows for displacement and subsequent dislocation or subluxation (Fig. 10). Characteristic radiographic findings are loss of vertebral height, and, occasionally, the presence of anterior chip fractures (teardrop fractures). Disruption of the posterior longitudinal ligament can be recognized if one carefully looks for widening of the spaces between the posterior spinous processes of the involved vertebral segments. Widening of the retropharyngeal space also is characteristically seen with compression fractures. Occasionally there may be associated spinous process or laminar fractures.[9,18]

Extreme care must be taken when diagnosing a compression fracture if there is no evidence of retropharyngeal widening, spinous process separation, or subluxation. Characteristically the infantile vertebral bodies have a wedge-shaped appearance that generally is replaced by the more normal vertebral body configuration by eight to ten years of age. This is not to be mistaken for a compression fracture.

With lower cervical spinal injuries in children, the degree of neurologic injury frequently is out of proportion to

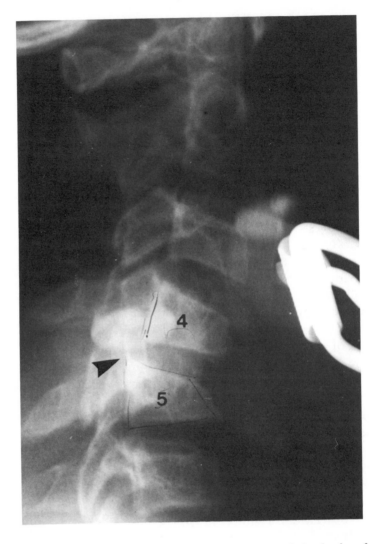

Figure 10. A typical compression fracture of the body of C5 associated with quadriplegia in a 16-year-old male. Note the associated disruption of the posterior longitudinal ligament that allows for displacement and subsequent dislocation and subluxation of C4-5 (arrow).

the extent of bony injury that is visualized radiographically. If this occurs, a careful radiological investigation, including plain tomograms, CT scans, myelography, or magnetic resonance imaging (MRI) is indicated.

THORACIC AND LUMBOSACRAL SPINAL FRACTURES

Only 5 percent of all cases of traumatic paraplegia secondary to thoracic or lumbar spine injuries occurs in children. Thoracic spinal injuries are relatively rare because of the intrinsic elasticity of the spine in this region as well as the stability provided by the rib cage. The most common type of fracture seen in both the thoracic and lumbosacral regions is the wedge or compression fracture. The mechanism of this type of injury is usually flexion, with or without associated rotation of the spine. The T4,T5 and L1,L2 levels are the most frequently affected levels in this type of injury.[12,16]

Careful radiological evaluation is often necessary to distinguish true wedge-compression fractures from normal vertebral body configurations in the child. Care also must be taken not to misinterpret the frequently seen vertical lucent cleft in the vertebral body as a fracture as this represents the nonossified neurocentral synchondrosis. Associated radiographic findings, which may be present with vertebral injury, are variations in spinal curvature characteristically occurring secondary to muscle spasm or ligamentous injury. Because of the intrinsic elasticity of the thoracic and lumbosacral spine, wedge fractures only rarely are associated with fractures of the posterior elements. Severe compression or burst of fractures, which are so commonly seen in adults, occur infrequently in children. When they do occur, CT scanning is helpful in delineating the presence of fragments within the spinal canal. Recently, MRI scanning has proved useful for direct visualization (Fig. 11) of the associated injury to the spinal cord or roots of the cauda equina (Fig. 12).[1,9]

As with lower cervical spinal fractures in children, it is not unusual for thoracic and lumbosacral fractures to have an associated neurologic deficit out of proportion to the radiographic findings.

SPINAL CORD INJURY WITHOUT RADIOGRAPHIC ABNORMALITY

In a young child, radiological diagnosis can be complicated by the extreme elasticity of the primarily cartilaginous

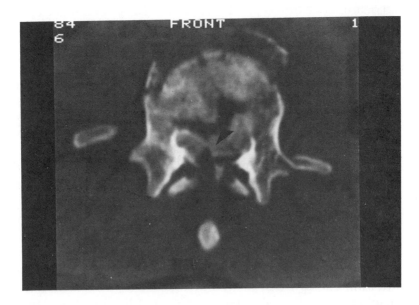

Figure 11. Computerized tomographic scan of the L1 vertebral body in a 15-year-old male who suffered a severe compression fracture with paraplegia. Multiple bony fragments almost completely obliterate the spinal canal (arrow).

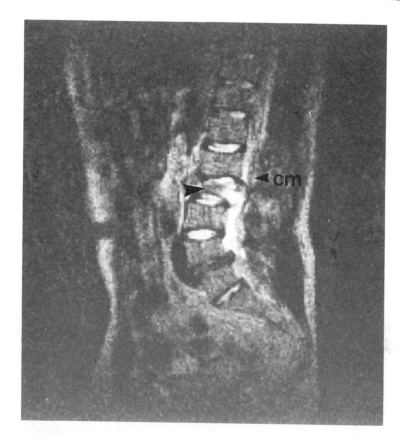

Figure 12. A magnetic resonance image of a 14-year-old with a severe compression fracture of L2 (arrow). The tip of the conus medularis (CM) is nicely visualized on the scan and indicates that the paraplegia is secondary to cauda equina rather than spinal cord injury.

spine and its supporting ligamentous structures. Such a situation can account for the occurrence of severe cord injury in the absence of any radiographic evidence of fracture or dislocation of the spine. The syndrome of spinal cord injury without radiographic abnormality (SCIWORA) has been estimated to occur in up to two-thirds of children with severe spine injuries under the age of eight. The mechanism of SCIWORA is poorly understood and may be related to severe hyperextension or flexion injuries with subsequent vascular compromise to the spinal cord, which results in ischemic injury or infarction of the cord. It is also possible, because of the extreme ligamentous laxity present in the pediatric spine, that severe degrees of subluxation may be allowed when trauma occurs. Subsequent rapid spontaneous reduction of this subluxation may result in mechanical injury to the cord and may produce neurologic deficits.[13]

In the presence of SCIWORA radiographic interpretation is extremely important. Should plain films fail to show any evidence of fracture, dislocation, or soft tissue injury, then it is important to obtain dynamic flexion-extension films. If any instability is present, it should be manifested by the occurrence of subluxation at the involved spinal level. Should plain radiographic films fail to show an abnormality in the presence of spinal cord injury, then it is essential to perform either biplane tomography or computerized axial tomography. Should these studies also prove normal, then myelography is indicated to rule out the presence of a subarachnoid block secondary to cord swelling. MRI scanning may prove useful in evaluation of the SCIWORA syndrome by allowing anatomical visualization of the spinal cord.

REFERENCES

1. Babcock JL: Spinal injuries in children. *Pediat Clin North Am* 22(2):487–501, 1975.
2. Ewald FC: Fracture of the odontoid process in a 17-month old infant treated with a halo. *J Bone Jt Surg* 53A(8):1636–1640, 1971.
3. Fielding JW, Hawkins RJ, Hensinger RN, Francis WR: Atlanto axial rotary deformities. *Orthop Clin North Am* 9(4):955–970, 1978.
4. Fielding JW, Hawkins RJ: Atlanto axial rotary fixation. *J Bone Jt Surg* 59A(1):37–44, 1977.
5. Gaufin LM, Goodman SJ: Cervical spine injuries in infants. *J Neurosurg* 42:179–182, 1975.

6. Gillis FH, Bina M, Soutrel A: Infantile atlanto occipital instability: The potential danger of extreme extension. *Am J Dis Child* 133:30–37, 1979.

7. Hachen HJ: Spinal cord injury in children and adolescents: Diagnostic pitfalls and therapeutic considerations in the acute stage. *Paraplegia* 15:55–64, 1977.

8. Griffiths SC: Fracture of the odontoid process in children. *J Pediat Surg* 6:680–685, 1972.

9. Heggenbarth R, Ebel KD: Roentgen findings in fractures of the vertebral column in children. *Pediatr Radiol* 5:34–39, 1976.

10. Marlin AE, Williams GR, Lee JF: Jefferson fractures in children. *J Neurosurg* 58:277–279, 1983.

11. McCrae DL: Significance of abnormalities of the cervical spine. *Am J Roentgenol* 84,(1):3–26, 1960.

12. Fielding JW: The cervical spine in the child, in O'Brien MS (ed): *Pediatric Neurological Surgery*. New York, Raven Press, 1978, pp 147–171.

13. Pang D, Wilberger JE: Spinal cord injury without radiographic abnormalities in children. *J Neurosurg* 57:114–129, 1982.

14. Pang D, Wilberger JE: Traumatic atlanto occipital dislocation with survival: Case report and review. *Neurosurg* 7:503–508, 1980.

15. Papavasilou V: Traumatic subluxation of the cervical spine during childhood. *Orthop Clin North America* 9(4):925–951, 1978.

16. Rang M (ed): Children's Fractures, ed 2. Toronto, J.B. Lippincott, 1974, pp 331–345.

17. Seimon LP: Fractures of the odontoid process in young children. *J Bone Jt Surg* 59A(7):943–948, 1977.

18. Sherk HH, Schut L, Lane JM: Fractures and dislocations of the cervical spine in children. *Orthop Clin North America* 7(3):593–604, 1976.

19. Teng P, Papatheodorou C: Traumatic subluxation of C2 in young children. *Bull Los Angeles Neurol Soc* 32:197–202, 1967.

20. Weiss MH, Kaufmann B: Hangman's fracture in an infant. *Am J Dis Child* 126:268–269, 1973.

Chapter 3

INITIAL ASSESSMENT AND NEUROLOGIC EVALUATION OF THE SPINAL CORD INJURED CHILD

Injury to the spine or spinal cord should be suspected in any unconscious child in whom there is evidence of multiple injuries or a significant head injury. From 5 percent to 20 percent of children with severe head injuries will have an associated cervical spine injury.[1,2] Additionally, any awake injured child who complains of numbness or weakness in the arms or legs or back or neck pain should be considered to have a spine and/or spinal cord injury until proven otherwise.

INITIAL MANAGEMENT OF SUSPECTED SPINAL CORD INJURY

Injuries sufficiently severe to cause spinal or spinal cord injury are characteristically associated with head, abdominal, or chest injuries. If such injuries coexist then immediate consideration should be given to treatment of those injuries that are most life-threatening. However, it should always be kept in mind that a multiply injured child may harbor a spinal cord injury, and it is best to assume this until neurologic examination proves otherwise.

In initial management, the establishment and maintenance of an airway is of primary importance. Often, multiply injured children will require intubation. Likewise, high level spinal cord injuries may cause acute respiratory embarrassment. With suspected spinal cord injury, any extension or manipulation of the neck is to be avoided. Therefore, when required, intubation is best achieved by the nasotracheal route.

Appropriate large bore intravenous lines must be established and appropriate fluid resuscitation started. If possible, a Foley catheter should be placed in the bladder.

Once initial stabilization is achieved, consideration must be given to transporting the child. The importance of proper management of the movement of the child with suspected spinal injury at the accident site cannot be overemphasized. Before any effort is made to move the child, some attempt should be made to ascertain whether there is movement in the arms or legs. Also, if the child is aware and old enough to cooperate, he should be asked about any neck or back pain or arm or leg numbness.

During transport from the scene of the injury to the emergency room, or from hospital to hospital, adequate stabilization of the entire spine is essential. A wooden or metal backboard, with the patient transported in the supine position, usually provides sufficient stabilization for any thoracic or lumbosacral spinal injuries. In small children, the neck can often be stabilized by taping the head to the backboard. Older children, particularly those who may be agitated secondary to head injury, are best stabilized by the use of sandbags and generous taping of the head (Fig. 1).

Vomiting is a frequent occurrence in injured children. Thus, if a child is to be transported in a supine position with the neck rigidly stabilized, insertion of a nasogastric tube is essential to prevent aspiration if vomiting occurs.

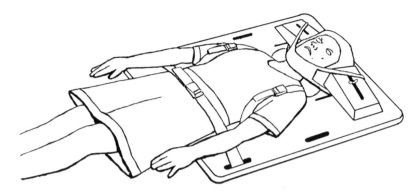

Figure 1. Immediate immobilization of the cervical spine is best accomplished by placing the child on a hard board, supporting the head with sandbags and taping or straps.

INITIAL ASSESSMENT FOR SPINAL CORD INJURY

Once stabilization has been achieved and other life-threatening injuries dealt with, initial assessment of a child suspected of having a spinal cord injury should consist of inspection and palpation and a careful determination of neurologic functioning, assuming that the child is not unconscious.[3,6]

Children with multiple injuries who have associated abrasions or lacerations on the face and forehead should be suspected of having a cervical hyperextension injury. Vertex scalp lacerations may be associated with cervical compression fractures. Children with abrasions of the upper neck may have suffered a flexion injury of the dorsal spine. A fracture of the mandible or associated contusion or abrasions about the jaw may have been associated with a rotational injury of the cervical spine. Bruises about the abdomen, as from a seat belt, may be associated with lumbar fractures.

Palpation of the spine is extremely important in the

initial evaluation. Local tenderness should always be carefully looked for, and if present, strongly suggests underlying bony, muscular, or ligamentous injury. A focal hematoma suggests a direct blow to the spine and may be associated with posterior element fractures. Widening of the spaces between two spinous processes suggests a significant ligamentous injury to the spine secondary to extreme flexion and may be associated with a compression fracture or subluxation of the spine.

The neurologic assessment of the awake child should not be difficult if some degree of cooperation can be established. A complete cord injury is generally associated with immediate loss of motor, reflex, and sensory function below the level of the lesion. Initial evaluation of motor function should seek to answer two questions (1) is the child able to voluntarily move the lower limbs and (2) is the child able to move his hands and fingers. Initial sensory exam should attempt to establish whether there is a relative loss of appreciation of painful sensation below a certain level on the trunk and to perform a careful testing of the sacral dermatomes. Sparing of sacral sensation, even if motor and reflex activity as well as other sensations are absent, may indicate that the degree of injury is not as severe as it initially appears. Such a situation deserves rapid diagnostic and corrective therapy. Similarly, important reflex activities to ascertain are the bulbocavernosus reflex and the anal wink reflex. Both reflexes involve sacral cord reflex pathways. Stimulation of the bulbocavernosus muscles by squeezing the base of the penis or the vulva should produce a reflex contraction of the internal anal sphincter. Similarly, painful stimulation of the skin around the anus should produce a reflex contraction of the external anal sphincter—the so-called anal wink. Presence of these reflexes indicates an incomplete cord lesion regardless of what the remainder of the examination may indicate.[6,7,14]

The problem of spinal shock often clouds the initial assessment of the spinal cord injured child. Spinal shock is a misunderstood term that can be used to denote two widely disparate problems. Spinal shock is often used in referring to the sympathetic vasomotor paralysis that can accompany severe cord injuries. This vasomotor paralysis results in hypotension, which may mimic the symptoms of shock secondary to blood loss. Spinal shock also is used to refer to the complete disappearance of all cord function below the level of injury. On occasion, spinal shock may simply represent a concussive injury to the cord with resultant return of function over a relatively rapid period of time. However, more often, spinal shock is associated with severe irreversible injury to the cord. With spinal shock, the bulbocavernosus reflex is characteristically absent. Return of this reflex heralds the end of spinal shock, and the resultant associated neurologic deficits are often permanent.[2,6]

In the unconscious child with an associated head injury, neurologic assessment is often difficult. The only clues to the presence of a significant spinal cord injury may be a lack of facial grimacing to peripherally applied pain, indicating a sensory loss over the trunk or a lack of withdrawal behaviors of the arms or the legs in response to painful stimulation of the head and face.

The importance of obtaining an accurate neurologic assessment cannot be overemphasized and serves a twofold purpose. Knowledge of the level of neurologic dysfunction is used to rationally plan the radiological studies needed to determine presence or absence of bony injury. Additionally, in children with incomplete spinal cord lesions, repeated neurologic examinations are extremely important and any deterioration in status requires aggressive intervention.

CLINICAL SYNDROMES ASSOCIATED WITH ACUTE CORD INJURY

Several characteristic syndromes have been described in association with spinal injuries. Spinal cord concussion was first described by Obersteiner in 1878.[2] A concussion can be said to have occurred after a "single violent impact to the vertebral column when the function of the spinal cord is affected though no gross anatomic changes can be found." If complete neurologic recovery occurs in a short period of time the injury is usually termed a spinal concussion. The "burning hands" syndrome of spinal cord injury was described by Maroon in 1977. In this syndrome, the only complaint is painful, burning dysesthesia in the hands and occasionally in the feet. There are few, if any, objective neurologic abnormalities. This syndrome can occur with or without an associated fracture or dislocation.[9,10] Both the spinal cord concussion and burning hands syndrome are much more common in the child than in the adult. The syndrome of complete cord transection results in immediate and sustained loss of all motor, reflex, and sensory modalities below the anatomical level of the lesion. This may occur because of complete physical anatomical disruption or complete physiological disruption of the cord (Fig. 2). The anterior spinal artery syndrome implies complete loss of cord function in the territory supplied by the anterior spinal artery. The anterior spinal artery provides nourishment to the anterior two-thirds of the spinal cord. Only the dorsal columns receive separate vascular supply. Thus, in the anterior spinal artery syndrome, preservation of function is limited to touch and proprioceptive sensations that are carried through the dorsal columns (Fig. 2). The Brown-Sequard syndrome involves a hemisection of the spinal cord with resultant loss of pain and temperature appreciation on the side opposite the lesion and all motor function on the side of and below the level of the lesion (Fig. 2). The central cord syndrome refers to an injury that is most severe in the center of the cord and less severe toward the periphery. Because of the somatotopic organization of the spinothalamic and corticospinal tracts, motor innervation of the arms is located centrally, while lumbosacral sensory modalities are located peripherally in the cord. In the

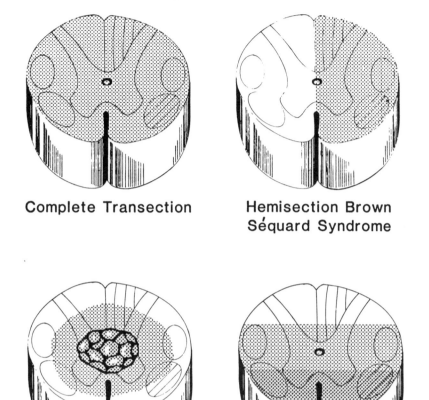

Complete Transection

**Hemisection Brown
Séquard Syndrome**

**Central Cord
Syndrome**

**Anterior Spinal
Artery Syndrome**

Figure 2. *Distribution of lesions that produce typical spinal cord syndromes.*

central cord syndrome, motor strength to the arms is more severely affected than that to the legs, while sacral sensation is often spared (Fig. 2).[13,14,15]

    The importance of delineating the clinical syndrome

associated with acute spinal cord injury lies in its prognostic significance. Complete cord transections and anterior spinal artery syndromes imply complete and permanent loss of all spinal cord function below the level of the injury with little chance for recovery. A Brown-Séquard syndrome implies a somewhat improved chance of recovery. Functional restitution of cord function has occurred in up to one-third of patients in whom the syndrome is present. The central cord syndrome has the best prognostic significance of all cord injuries. Two-thirds of patients with this syndrome will have a significant degree of functional recovery.

When confronted with spinal injuries and associated neurologic dysfunction, it must be kept in mind that the spinal cord level and the vertebral level do not correspond. In the cervical region, the cord level is about one segment higher than the corresponding vertebral level, i.e., the C3 cord level lies opposite the C2 vertebral body and spinous process. In the lower cervical and thoracic region, there is a difference of approximately two levels, while in the lumbar region there is a three-segment discrepancy. By one year of age the spinal cord usually terminates at the L1-2 vertebral level. Thus, an injury to the sacral spinal cord can result from an L1 fracture (Fig. 3). The typical motor and sensory findings associated with various levels of spinal cord injury are outlined below (Figs. 4 and 5).[5,11]

C1 through C4

An injury to the spinal cord at the level of C1 to C4 results in complete paralysis of all voluntary movement in the trunk and limbs. A C2 injury results in loss of sensation up to the vertex of the head where the V1 trigeminal distribution begins. A C4 injury results in loss of sensation to slightly above the level of the clavicle. Often, because of the supraclavicular nerves (C2,C3 innervation), which extend below the level of the clavicle, it appears that sensation is preserved down to the nipple line when a C4 level injury is

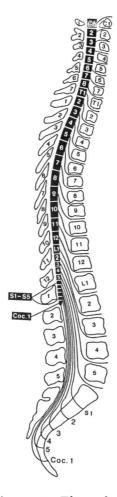

Figure 3. The relationship of the spinal cord
segments and nerve roots
to the vertebral bodies.
Note that the spinal cord
ends at the L1-2 vertebral
level.

present. The possibility of supraclavicular innervation must
be recognized so as not to create confusion regarding the
level of the lesion. The extreme importance of C1 to C4 level

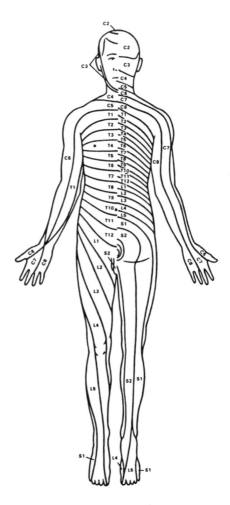

Figure 4. Dermatomal chart
showing the typical segmental
sensory distribution.

lesions is that they result not only in the denervation of all
respiratory muscles but in bilateral paralysis of the diaphragm as well. Many patients with this level lesion will
not survive because of associated respiratory distress. If
they do survive, then they are often ventilator dependent.

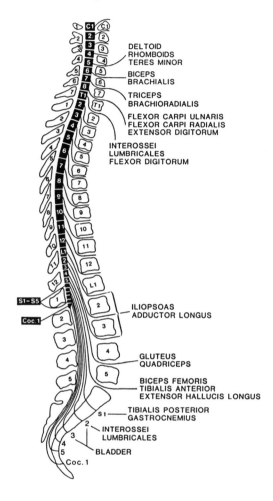

DELTOID
RHOMBOIDS
TERES MINOR

BICEPS
BRACHIALIS

TRICEPS
BRACHIORADIALIS

FLEXOR CARPI ULNARIS
FLEXOR CARPI RADIALIS
EXTENSOR DIGITORUM

INTEROSSEI
LUMBRICALES
FLEXOR DIGITORUM

ILIOPSOAS
ADDUCTOR LONGUS

GLUTEUS
QUADRICEPS

BICEPS FEMORIS
TIBIALIS ANTERIOR
EXTENSOR HALLUCIS LONGUS

TIBIALIS POSTERIOR
GASTROCNEMIUS

INTEROSSEI
LUMBRICALES

BLADDER

Figure 5. Distribution of segmental muscle innervation.

C5

An injury to the spinal cord at the level of C5 results in denervation of all voluntary muscles below the level of the deltoids. Thus, the only movements that the patient is capable of are movement of the neck and possibly weak abduction of the arms. With a C5 lesion, the diaphragm is only partially denervated although the remainder of the respiratory muscles are paralyzed. With such an injury, it is often possible for the patient to sustain an independent respiratory effort with minimal assistance. C5 lesions produce impaired sensory function over the entire body with the exception of the lateral arm and forearm.

C6

With a C6 level lesion, the only muscles that are spared denervation and paralysis are the deltoid, biceps, and brachioradialis muscles. All hand, trunk, and lower limb muscles are paralyzed. While there may be a transient impairment of diaphragmatic function with a C6 level lesion, this usually returns to normal after the period of spinal shock subsides. Because of the uninhibited contraction of the spared muscle groups with a C6 lesion, these children often have a characteristic posture with the shoulders elevated, the arms abducted, and the forearms flexed. Sensation is intact down to the level of the upper arm and forearm with a C6 level lesion.

C7

With a C7 lesion, elbow extension, pronation of the forearm, flexion of the wrist, and extension of the fingers are all impaired because of denervation of the triceps, flexor carpi radialis, and extensor digitorum communis. Patients will retain voluntary control over the deltoid, biceps, and brachioradialis, allowing them to elevate their arms and bend the elbow. Diaphragmatic function is left intact as is use of accessory respiratory muscles in spite of loss of intercostal and abdominal muscle function. With a C7 level lesion, sensation should be intact down through the thumb, index, and possibly the middle fingers.

C8

With a C8 level lesion, some minimal degree of wrist function is preserved. Voluntary muscle denervation includes the flexor carpi ulnaris, flexor digitorum sublimus, and flexor digitorum profundus, which results in significant impairment in finger function. Respiration is only minimally affected because of intercostal abdominal muscle denervation. Sensation is spared through the middle and ring fingers when a C8 level lesion is present.

T1

Injury at the T1 cord segment results in denervation of all the voluntary muscles of the intrinsic hand, as well as all trunk and lower extremity muscles. Preserved are functions of the upper arm and wrist flexion and extension. Respiratory function is not severely affected. Sensation in a C8 level lesion is intact in the hand and into the lower aspect of the medial forearm.

Thoracic Level

Injuries to the thoracic cord result in paraplegia with a varying degree of associated intercostal and abdominal muscle denervation. This generally produces respiratory problems only with extreme degrees of stress. Several landmarks of sensory perception should be kept in mind when dealing with thoracic cord injuries. The T4 sensory level corresponds to the nipple line, the T10 sensory level corresponds to the umbilicus, and T12 sensation is slightly above the level of the inguinal ligament. The thoracic cord injuries characteristically result in loss of sacral sensation as well as bowel and bladder function.

Conus Injuries

The conus lies at the level of the L1 and L2 vertebral bodies. The conus is the terminal portion of the spinal cord representing the majority of lumbar and sacral outflow. Thus, a spinal injury at the L1-L2 level will result in a conus injury that is equivalent to a low spinal cord injury. With conus lesions, sensation is usually affected in a saddle distribution with bilateral symmetrical loss of sensation in the sacral region. Sacral sensory loss is accompanied by bowel and bladder dysfunction. Lumbar sensory loss may occur up to the L1 or L2 level (inguinal ligament or thigh). In a complete conus lesion paraplegia is usually present.

Cauda Equina

Cauda equina injuries generally result from bony injuries below the level of L2. Because the roots of the cauda equina are peripheral nerves, prognosis for recovery from such injury is generally quite good.[12] Depending on the roots that are injured, a variety of neurologic findings may be present. These findings are characteristically asymmetrical in their sensory and motor manifestations. Bowel and bladder function may be spared depending on the roots that are injured.

SPECIAL PROBLEMS OF THE SPINAL CORD INJURED CHILD

Spinal Shock

Immediately following a severe spinal cord injury, the child will develop spinal shock, a term introduced in 1850 by Hall.[7] Spinal shock refers to the complete suppression of all reflex, motor, and sensory activity that follows any physiological or anatomical injury to the cord. The modern concept of spinal shock is based on the work of Sherrington, who postulated that a transient depression in the segments below the spinal cord injury occurs due to a sudden withdrawal of the predominantly facilitating influences of descending supraspinal tracts from higher centers. This results in disruption of transmission at the synapse level.[3,6,11]

The most obvious sign of spinal shock, evident to the patient as well as the examiner, is the motor paralysis below the level of the lesion. Paralysis is at first flaccid, but if it is of an upper motor neuron type, there will be reflex return once the spinal shock has subsided. During the state of spinal shock all reflexes, both cutaneous and deep, below the level of the lesion are depressed or abolished. In children, spinal shock usually lasts less than one week. In adults, this may persist up to six weeks. Once spinal shock disappears, reflex responses begin to reappear. The first returning reflexes are the anal and bulbocavernosus reflexes and response to plantar stimulation with withdrawal of the foot. Once spinal shock is resolved, the remaining neurologic function usually will persist throughout the life of the child.

Neurogenic spinal shock must be differentiated from vasomotor spinal shock. In the latter instance, there is an associated drop in blood pressure, which may be quite dramatic. This results from sympathetic vascular denervation with subsequent vasodilatation producing a shocklike picture. In the patient who is multiply injured, it is sometimes difficult to determine whether the low blood pressure is secondary to associated blood loss or related to the spinal injury. In the case of blood loss producing shock, pressure can often be maintained by using mast trousers on the lower extremities or by adequate fluid resuscitation. With spinal vasomotor shock, fluid resuscitation is often ineffective because of the abnormal vascular tone, and vasopressors are often necessary for adequate restoration of a normal blood pressure.

Respiratory Problems

The reduction in early mortality from spinal cord injury is, for the most part, related to improvements in respiratory care. The problems of pulmonary insufficiency secondary to the neurologic lesion are often compounded by direct injuries to the chest and lung parenchyma as well as by the aspiration of blood or vomitus, the latter pointing out the necessity for early placement of a nasogastric tube to empty the stomach of its contents. With high cervical cord lesions and severely compromised diaphragmatic function, vital capacity may drop to 0.1 to 0.3 L. In children with even the slightest cervical spinal cord injury, careful observation of the ventilatory pattern is imperative. If hypoventilation, irregular breathing, sighing, or unexplained air hunger occurs, even in the presence of normal arterial blood gases, endotracheal intubation and mechanical ventilation is indicated. Controlled respiration is usually necessary for less than one week.

Phrenic nerve dysfunction occurs with high cervical cord injuries, resulting in loss of diaphragmatic excursion, which may be unilateral or bilateral. In such a situation the child cannot survive without mechanical ventilation.

Autonomic Dysfunction

When the spinal cord is severely injured, regulatory autonomic impulses from the cerebral cortex, brain stem, and intermediolateral columns of the spinal cord are interrupted and various types of dysfunction occur. If the spinal cord is interrupted above the T9 level, heat-induced sweating is lost below the level of the lesion. If the injury is above C8, all thermoregulatory impulses from the hypothalamus are blocked, and no sweating in response to outside temperature is possible. However, severe reflex sweating may occur secondary to significant bladder or rectal distension. It is important to recognize this phenomenon as a severe temperature regulatory dysfunction may develop with lack of sweating. If the ambient temperature is warm, then the child is unable to dissipate heat through sweating and the core body temperature may rise. Similarly, if excessive sweating occurs secondary to a bladder or rectal distension, fluid loss may be increased considerably in the small child. As noted in the description of spinal shock, sympathetic vasomotor control is significantly affected by a complete spinal cord lesion. Occasionally as a result of this paralytic vessel dilitation, the nasopharyngeal mucosa is swollen and blockage of the air passages may result. This is extremely important to consider when respiratory function is already compromised by a high cervical injury. Once the acute phase of vasogenic spinal shock wears off, blood pressure control presents no significant problem. However, it must be kept in mind that orthostatic hypotension will occur rapidly if the child's position is changed toward the vertical as the compensatory vascular constrictive reflexes are lost.[8,11]

Loss of autonomic control also results in an inability to regulate heart rate. Because of uninhibited vagal tone, bradycardia is extremely common in the initial stages of spinal cord injury. The bradycardia can be so profound as to require treatment with atropine or placement of a temporary pacemaker. Also because of the sympathetic outflow injury, the gastrointestinal tract becomes hypotonic or atonic. This can result in gastric distension, subsequent vomiting, and potential for aspiration and serves to further emphasize the need for rapid placement of nasogastric tubes for gastric emptying. A prolonged ileus may result following a spinal cord injury, and characteristically the reflexes controlling defecation also are abolished. Significant abdominal distension from paralytic ileus may further compromise respiratory function by causing elevation of the diaphragm.

Bladder Dysfunction

With a complete spinal cord injury, the bladder initially cannot respond to distension as the somatic muscles are flaccid. Since the bladder is innervated through an automatic intramural network, which provides inherent elasticity, complete atony does not occur. It is important to realize that bladder distension may occur rapidly following spinal cord injuries, and this distension may set off undesirable autonomic reflexes, which can result in hypotension or bradycardia. Thus, when dealing with the spinal cord injured child, it is important to rapidly insert a Foley catheter to prevent subsequent bladder distension.[8]

REFERENCES

1. Babcock JL: Spinal injuries in children. *Pediat Clin North Am* 22:487–500, 1975.
2. Braakman R, Penning L: Injuries of the cervical spine, in Vinken PJ, Bruyn GW (eds): *Handbook of Clinical Neurology, Injuries of the Spine and Spinal Cord, Part 1*. Amsterdam, North Holland, 1976, vol 25, pp 227–380.
3. Bumpus HC, Nourse MH, Thompsons GJ: Neurologic complications in injury of the spinal cord. *JAMA* 133:366, 1947.
4. Burk DC: Spinal trauma in children. *Paraplegia* 9:1–14, 1971.
5. Crosby E, Humphrey T, Louer E: *Correlative Anatomy of the Nervous System*. New York, Macmillan Co, 1972, pp 1–79.
6. Geisler WO, Wynne-Jones M, Jousse AT: Early management of patients with trauma to the spinal cord. *Med J Canada* 22:512–523, 1966.
7. Hachen HJ: Spinal cord injuries in children and adolescents: Diagnostic pitfalls and therapeutic considerations in the acute state. *Paraplegia* 15:55–64, 1977.
8. Head H, Riddock G: The autonomic bladder, excessive sweating and some other reflex conditions in gross injuries of the spinal cord. *Pain* 40:188, 1917.
9. Maroon, JC: "Burning Hands" in football spinal cord injuries. *JAMA* 238:2049–2051.
10. Maroon JC, Steele PB, Berlin R: Football head and neck injuries—an update. *Clin Neurosurg* 27:414–429, 1980.
11. Ogden JA: *Skeletal Injury in the Child*. Philadelphia, Lea & Febiger, 1982, pp 385–423.

12. Ransohff J: Lesions of the cauda equina. *Clin Neurosurg* 17:331–344, 1970.
13. Schneider RD: The syndrome of acute anterior spinal cord injury. *J Neurosurg* 12:95–122, 1955.
14. Schneider RD, Cherry G, Pantack H: The syndrome of acute cervical spinal cord injury: Special reference to the mechanism involved in hyperextension injuries of the cervical spine. *J Neurosurg* 11:547–577, 1954.
15. Schneider RD, Crosby EC, Russo RH, Gosch HH: Traumatic spinal cord syndromes and their management. *Clin Neurosurg* 20:424, 1973.

Chapter 4

CLINICAL ASPECTS OF SPECIFIC SPINAL INJURIES

As the patterns of spinal injuries are different from children to adults, the clinical aspects of various fractures and dislocations that may have a common anatomical basis are often markedly different. The characteristic and at times unique clinical aspects of these various injuries in children must be understood to effectively direct the radiological diagnosis and appropriate treatment.

SPINAL IMMOBILIZATION

The first and foremost principle in the management of known spinal injury with or without associated spinal cord injury is immobilization of the spine and reduction of any associated dislocations. Initial immobilization and reduction is best achieved by skeletal traction. Many devices are available for skeletal traction, the most popular are the Gardner-Wells (GW) tongs (Fig. 1). The GW tongs consist of a pair of spring-loaded pins that can be directly applied to the skull through the scalp in a matter of minutes. They can be positioned to allow for traction in flexion, extension, or neutral position, depending on the type of dislocation that is present. Older skull traction devices such as the Crutchfield, Vinke, or Blackburn tongs generally have been aban-

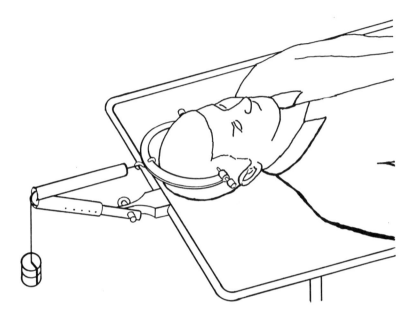

Figure 1. *Gardner-Wells tongs provide the most stable initial form of immobilization for cervical spinal injuries.*

doned because they require placement of burr holes for their attachment. Increasing use is being made of the halo ring for skull traction. Placement of the halo ring is similar to that of the GW tongs, however, four pins are used to fix the device to the skull.[11]

These devices generally can be used in children over two years of age. However, in children less than 18 months of age, the skull may not be sufficiently thick to allow for skull traction devices. In such a situation, some have advocated placing two burr holes on opposite sides of the skull through which wire can be passed and connected to traction. In many cases, however, in very young children immobilization can be maintained simply by taping the head to the bed or other similar external devices.[7]

Generally, skull traction devices should only be placed by those experienced in their management. Weights can be applied subsequently to the traction to aid in realignment of the spine. It is recommended that no more than 5 lb of weight be applied for each cervical level involved—i.e., for a C6 level dislocation no more than 30 lb of weight should be used. With the proper amount of weight and the appropriate degree of associated flexion or extension, reduction of most dislocations in children can be achieved (Fig. 2).

If reduction cannot be achieved with traction some have advocated closed reduction or manipulation of the neck. While this is apparently a standard practice in Europe and Australia with no reported neurologic worsening, the chances for causing vascular or further spinal cord injury with manipulation are considerable.

SPINAL CORD CONCUSSION/ BURNING HANDS SYNDROME

Spinal cord concussion implies a reversible physiological derangement in cord function resulting from the transmission of force to the spinal cord without associated direct spinal injury. Transient synaptic dysfunction may occur secondary to alterations in membrane potentials, neurotransmitter availability, or microcirculatory abnormalities. Various types of neurologic abnormalities may occur in association with spinal cord concussion, ranging from complete loss of all function to mild nerve root symptoms. Fortunately, all associated neurologic dysfunction completely disappears in a short period of time (usually less than one hour). However, even when symptoms and findings resolve, it is imperative to perform a complete workup to rule out the possibility of bony injury. Observation in the hospital for at least 24 hours or until all symptoms resolve is indicated.

The burning hands syndrome was first described in conjunction with athletic neck injury but subsequently has been found to be increasingly common in children. The

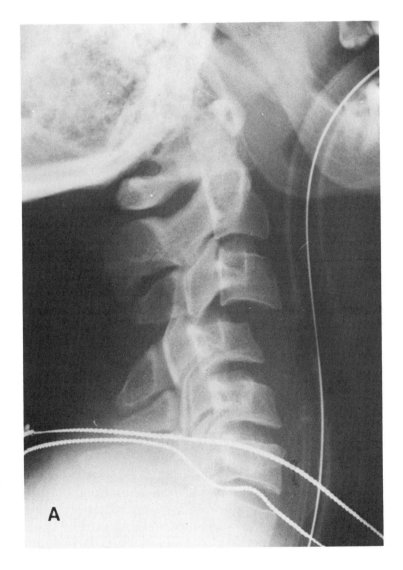

Figure 2A. *A severe dislocation at the C3-4 level associated with quadriplegia in a 15-year-old boy involved in an automobile accident.*

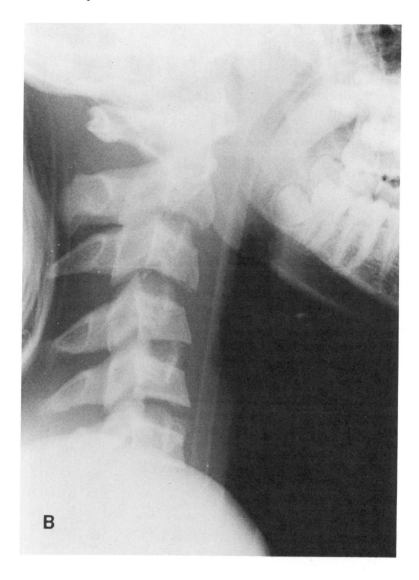

Figure 2B. *After application of Gardner-Wells tongs and 30 lbs of traction, the dislocation is almost completely reduced. Using the Gardner-Wells tongs, the spine can be maintained in this position until fusion is performed.*

syndrome is characterized by burning dysesthesia in the hands and fingertips and occasionally in the feet. Pathologically, this syndrome is felt to result from a mild central cord injury. Recently, with magnetic resonance imaging, abnormalities in the cord have been identified (Fig. 3). Characteristically the burning sensation lasts for 18 to 24 hours before dissipating. The presence of this syndrome requires careful workup to rule out associated bony injury as up to 50 percent of children with this complaint will be found to have a cervical fracture or dislocation. If no bony abnormalities are found then in-hospital observation is indicated until symptoms resolve.

ATLANTO-OCCIPITAL DISLOCATION

Traumatic atlanto-occipital (A-O) dislocation rarely is recognized clinically. Only 13 cases have been reported in the world literature with only seven patients surviving this

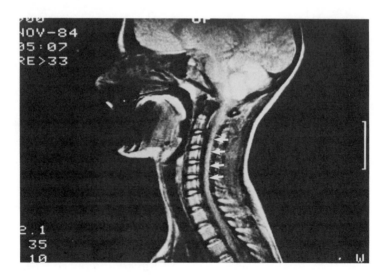

Figure 3. A magnetic resonance image of the cervical spinal cord in a 12-year-old girl with burning hands syndrome. Arrows outline the area of cord contusion from C2 to C4.

type of injury. Of the 13 cases recorded, nine patients were less than 18 years of age. The reason that this type of injury is not frequently recognized is that more often than not A-O dislocation results in total cervicomedullary dislocation with subsequent respiratory arrest and death.[13]

Lesser degrees of damage to the lower brain stem and upper cervical cord may become evident as cardiorespiratory instability with associated brachycardia, irregular respirations, or apnea. Cranial nerve palsies as well as other brain stem signs have been seen in association with A-O dislocation. Findings such as rotary nystagmus, ocular bobbing, decerebrate posturing, and lower cranial nerve dysfunction have all been recognized in patients with this injury. Flaccid quadriplegia, hemiparesis and Brown-Séquard syndrome have all been seen in patients with A-O dislocation. Similarly, the presence of a Horner's syndrome has also been reported.[8]

Since it is felt that the most likely mechanism of atlanto-occipital dislocation is extreme hyperextension in association with lateral flexion, an alerting sign to the possibility of the presence of such an injury is the presence of abrasions, lacerations, or contusions involving the chin or lateral aspects of the face.

The initial treatment of suspected atlanto-occipital dislocation requires complete immobilization of the head. Generally, when a cervical spine injury is suspected, skeletal traction is employed as a means of providing immediate immobilization. However, if A-O dislocation is present, placement of weights with distraction of the neck may result in significant worsening of the neurologic status. Thus, it has been advocated that once the clinical and neurologic diagnosis has been established, the patient's head should be immobilized by the use of the halo apparatus. As A-O dislocation primarily involves ligamentous injury, it is an extremely unstable injury on a long-term basis. Thus, once the immediate complications associated with the injury are stabilized, it is recommended that atlanto-occipital axial fusion be performed (Fig. 4).

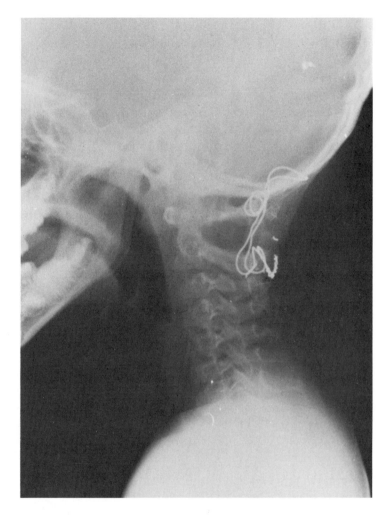

Figure 4. An occipito-atlanto-axial fusion has been performed in this 5-year-old girl who suffered atlanto-occipital dislocation with an associated Brown-Séquard syndrome.

ATLAS FRACTURES

Atlas or Jefferson's fractures are rare in children. When they do occur, they rarely are associated with significant spinal cord injury. As the mechanism of injury is generally axial compression, the fracture essentially represents a bursting fracture of the ring of C1 with centripetal displacement of the fragments.[19]

In one reported case of a Jefferson's fracture in a three-year-old child, the main symptom was an inability to hold the head in an upright position with the child complaining of a sense of instability of the neck. However, in other reported cases, the only symptoms noted were those of neck pain frequently associated with cervical muscle spasm and torticollis. The neurologic examination is generally normal.[10]

Because the injury involves the bone rather than ligamentous structures, the preferred mode of treatment is immobilization of the spine to allow bony union to occur. For children over two years of age, the halo apparatus is the preferred method of immobilization. For younger children, the halo has been modified to include a skullcap and a plastic jacket to provide immobilization with good results. A Minerva jacket is sometimes necessary to achieve good immobilization. Immobilization is often necessary for three to four months to achieve satisfactory bony union.

ATLANTOAXIAL SUBLUXATION

Isolated C1-C2 dislocation occurs secondary to rupture of the transverse dental ligament. Traumatic rupture of this ligament is rare because the more vulnerable dens usually fails before the ligament ruptures resulting in an odontoid fracture. However, it is not infrequently seen to result secondary to inflammations such as tonsillitis or pharyngitis and is at times associated with juvenile rheumatoid arthritis. Failure of this ligament allows for the dislocation of C1 on C2 with the atlas sliding anteriorly and subsequent narrowing of the diameter of the spinal canal at the C2 level. The presenting symptom with a traumatic C1-C2 subluxation is usually an isolated complaint of torticollis. In the most common type of displacement, the head is turned away from the affected side and neck movements are limited. However, with traumatic C1-C2 subluxation, if there is sufficient narrowing of the spinal canal a severe high-level spinal cord injury can result with associated respiratory distress.[19]

Because the injury is primarily ligamentous in nature, prolonged immobilization has little effect on the ultimate stability at the C1-C2 level. For this reason, C1-C2 fusion is often necessary to prevent progressive subluxation and spinal cord impingement.

ATLANTOAXIAL ROTARY SUBLUXATION

Rotary subluxation at the C1-C2 joint is a relatively common problem, particularly in children. It is primarily a ligamentous strain that results in a unilateral dislocation at the C1-C2 joint. It also can occur in association with upper respiratory infections, tonsillitis, pharyngitis, and similar conditions that may produce hyperemia in the upper cervical region. This can result in ligamentous laxity and instability of the C1-C2 joint.[6]

However, most often, rotary subluxation is produced by minor trauma. The characteristic story of such a trauma is one in which the child is wearing a billed cap that is twisted in play by another child, suddenly rotating and twisting the neck beyond its normal range. Subsequently, the child presents with a painful torticollis accompanied by marked spasm in the sternocleidomastoid muscle. The torticollis may take from 12 to 24 hours to develop subsequent to the injury. On examination, in addition to the obvious torticollis, there is usually tenderness over the sternocleidomastoid muscle as well as local tenderness over the C1-C2 joint when the posterior aspect of the neck is palpated.

Rotary subluxations at the atlantoaxial joint are usually temporary and are generally easily corrected. Treatment consists of hospitalization with continuous traction using a head halter and 3 to 5 lb of weights. Muscle relaxants are useful. With traction, the subluxation usually is spontaneously reduced within a few days with subsequent resolution of the muscle spasm. After reduction is complete, the patient's neck should be supported with a soft collar for several weeks and the child should not perform strenuous activities.

In extremely severe cases of rotary subluxation that are not corrected by halter traction, skeletal traction with tongs is sometimes necessary to achieve reduction. Occasionally, the ligamentous disruption is so severe that the joint remains unstable in spite of the reduction and atlantoaxial fusion is necessary.

An entity of atlantoaxial rotary fixation also has been described in which the subluxation was impossible to correct with traction or recurred when traction was stopped. This represents a much more severe entity with the potential for significant spinal cord injury if not corrected. The cause of this fixation is not known but may represent a type of locked facet with articular surface damage. Early atlantoaxial fusion is recommended in such cases.

AXIS FRACTURES

Dens Fractures

Fracture of the odontoid process is rare in children who are less than seven years old. It is even more rare in children less than three years old. In the majority of instances, fractures of the odontoid process in children are associated with major trauma and most of the fractures are readily diagnosed on the basis of early x-ray films. However, there is no diagnostic clinical syndrome associated with a fracture of the dens. The symptoms and signs may be so few and so indefinite that the diagnosis is missed. Characteristically, when the dens is fractured, pain is present that usually is severe and often referred to the occipital region. This may be accentuated in any attempt to move the head. The classic picture is that of the child who is supporting his head with his hands in order to prevent the slightest movement. The neck may be held twisted due to an associated torticollis. Occasionally, there may be minimal pain associated with a dens fracture, however, the child may resist any movement of the head without complaining bitterly. Palpation of the dens through the posterior pharynx will always produce pain if a fracture is present. However, this may be a very difficult undertaking in small children.[5,9,17,18]

The most common neurologic complication secondary to fracture of the dens is injury to the greater occipital nerve, which results in referred pain and occasional numbness over the occiput. Obviously, the most serious complication is the potential for upper spinal cord or lower brain stem compression from posterior displacement of the fractured dens process.

Treatment in most cases of fractures of the dens should be conservative with strict bed rest, initial skeletal traction, and subsequent cervical brace or halo cast. It is felt that dens fractures in children are similar to epiphyseal separations in other parts of the body in that they will unite readily and heal firmly once their position is reestablished and immobilization is achieved. With markedly displaced lesions with or without associated neurologic deficits, treatment may have to be modified. In older children and teenagers, the dental synchondrosis is fused with the body of C2 and injuries occurring in this age group must be treated the same as in adults. Generally, basilar and apical fractures of the dens heal well when reduced and stabilized, whereas fractures above the level of the atlantoaxial facets tend to remain unstable and often require operative fusion (Fig. 5).

The anteriorly displaced dens fracture in children can usually be reduced easily by gentle manipulation into extension with cervical skeletal traction. The ease of reduc-

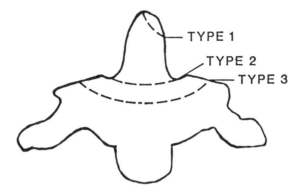

Figure 5. *Type I (apical) and type III (basalar)*
fractures of the dens generally heal well when
reduced and stabilized. Type II fractures across
the base of the odontoid process generally re-
quire operative fusion.

tion, stability with traction or halo support, early callus
formation, and prompt healing in most cases offer a good
prognosis in these patients, and surgical reduction or fusion
is rarely necessary. Although there is a high incidence (approximately 30 percent) of pseudoarthrosis or avascular
necrosis of dens fractures in adults, this does not seem to be
a serious complication in skeletally immature patients. Undisplaced fractures at the base of the dens within the substance of the body of the axis have a satisfactory potential
for healing and probably could be treated conservatively in
children with a stiff collar.

However, nonunion of dens fractures in children has
been described and this is felt to be the primary mechanism
for the development of an os odontoideum. Nonunion of the
fracture with subsequent fibrous replacement of the bone
has been documented in several children under five years
old. It also is well known that fractures through cartilaginous plates in other parts of the body will result in nonunion unless adequate immobilization is achieved. For this
reason, in a child, x-ray films should be obtained about four

months after suspected or definite dens fracture in order to demonstrate whether union has occurred. In three reported cases in children in whom dens injury was not recognized and treated, resorption of the basilar portion of the dens occurred that produced the appearance of congenital absence of the dens in one instance and of an os odontoideum in the other two. Thus, late atlantoaxial instability may complicate even a minimally displaced dens fracture and follow-up must be accurate and maintained until the child stops growing.

Hangman's Fracture

Fracture dislocation of the second cervical vertebrae with or without concomitant spinal cord injury is a rare occurrence in young children. In the hangman's fracture, cervical spine radiographs characteristically show a fracture of the pedicles of C2 with anterior subluxation of C1 and the body of C2 on C3. Because of the width of the spinal canal at the C2,C3 level and the nature of the injury with associated bursting type of fracture little spinal cord injury results. However, one case of a 12-month-old infant with a hangman's fracture has been reported in which a central cord injury resulted. If the neurologic examination is normal, the only clue to this injury may be local tenderness of the upper cervical spine with associated muscle spasms and neck stiffness.[19,22]

Because there is little ligamentous damage associated with most hangman's fractures in the adult, this lesion generally is properly treated by immobilization in a brace or halo cast for 8 to 12 weeks to allow spontaneous healing. However, the same lesion in an infant poses added therapeutic considerations because of the marked instability of the cervical spine at its early stage of development. In the only two cases reported in infants under the age of two years, presence of a hangman's fracture was associated with considerable instability of the upper cervical spine. In each case, an internal operative stabilization was required in order to ensure bony union.

Lower Cervical Spinal Fractures

Compression fractures of the lower cervical spine, with or without associated dislocation, are the most commonly seen injuries in children. The occurrence of unilateral or bilateral facet dislocations, which are the most common type of lower cervical spinal injury in adults, are not seen in children. A compression fracture of the lower cervical spine, occurring secondary to axial loading and hyperflexion injury, may be associated with any of the neurologic syndromes usually described for spinal cord injuries— complete cord transection, anterior cord syndrome, Brown-Séquard syndrome, central cord syndrome, burning hands syndrome, or a normal neurologic examination.[7,14,19]

When no dislocation or subluxation is present and the degree of bony compression is less than 25 percent of the expected vertebral body height, the symptoms are generally mild and often limited to pain on neck movements with associated muscle spasm. Treatment in such instances is generally symptomatic with a hard collar or cervical brace used to provide support until healing occurs.

When there is associated dislocation, ligamentous stability has been compromised. In adults, this almost always dictates operative fusion of the injury site. However, in children, if the degree of bony compression is not severe and the dislocation can be easily reduced by skeletal traction, the prognosis for stable healing is quite good with immobilization alone. The younger the child, the better the prognosis for spontaneous healing. In such a situation, the halo cast has proved quite successful and has been used in infants as young as 17 months. Stability at the fracture site is restored by ligamentous and osseous healing if the neck is held immobile in a reduced position. In young adolescents, however, spontaneous fusion is less likely and surgical fusion is often necessary (Fig. 6).

When a compression fracture is treated conservatively, careful radiological follow-up must be undertaken even if stable healing occurs. A fracture through the centrum of the vertebral body may result in a growth disturbance of the entire spinal segment. As a result of this, progressive kyphotic deformities may occur, giving rise to a worsening of a preexisting neurologic deficit or development of new neurologic problems. A child with such a fracture is at risk for such problems until all active growth has ceased. Therefore radiographs should be obtained at regular intervals until adolescence has passed.

Another potential complication of cervical compression fractures is acute disc herniation. This may result in a radicular pain syndrome with or without neurologic deficit. If the symptoms are not relieved by neck immobilization then further investigation including myelography is indicated.

Thoracic and Thoracolumbar Fractures

Injury to the spine in the thoracic region is rare in children due to the intrinsic elasticity of the spine in this region, coupled with the protective effect of the rib cage, which prevents excessive movements and protects from abnormal stresses that could produce fracture or dislocation. In the thoracic region, especially in younger children, injury to the spinal cord occurs more often without associated vertebral fractures.[21]

Minor wedge fractures of the vertebral bodies are relatively common and usually multiple. Because of the intrinsic elasticity of the thoracic spine in children, these injuries can occur without major damage to the posterior elements,

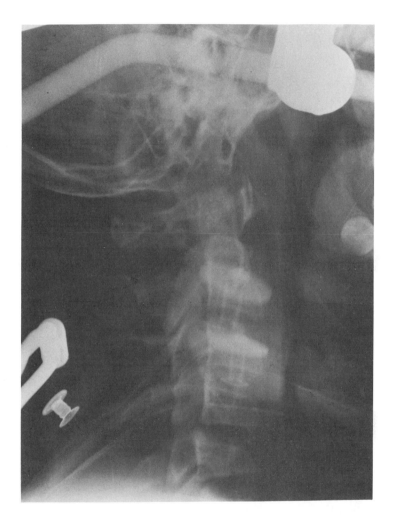

Figure 6. A C5 compression fracture in an 11-year-old following a diving accident. The posterior displacement at C5 indicates some degree of ligamentous instability. In this instance, after a trial of immobilization in a halo, spontaneous fusion did not occur and cervical fusion was necessary.

producing an intrinsically more stable injury than is seen in adults with similar fractures. The posterior and anterior longitudinal ligaments are usually not affected in simple wedge-compression fractures.

Thoracic compression fractures result from hyperflexion injuries. In children, multiple thoracic fractures are common because of healthy intervertebral discs, which can transmit the force from one vertebral body to the other. With simple compression or wedge fractures, physical examination is generally normal except for localized spine tenderness with or without associated muscle spasm. The occurrence of spinal cord injury in association with a simple compression fracture is quite rare.[2]

Important information as to the ability of these wedge fractures to heal spontaneously comes from the series by Ruckstuhl who studied a total of 65 thoracic vertebral fractures in children. If the wedge fractures show a deformity of the bone in the sagittal plane, only then is the prognosis for spontaneous healing better than if the bony deformity is evident in the frontal plane as well. Those children with only sagittal deformities tend to show a restoration of vertebral height during subsequent growth, but improvement in the wedge deformity occurs in only one-third of children with a frontal plane deformity. If the endplates are fractured as well as the body, then no correction of the deformity can occur spontaneously.[15]

Rotation or flexion-rotation forces characteristically produce the most severe and unstable thoracic or thoracolumbar fractures (Fig. 7). The majority of these injuries are the result of automobile accidents. Such injuries often result in posterior element fractures, vertebral compression fractures, and combination fracture-dislocations. Approximately 50 percent of children with such injuries will have an associated neurologic deficit in the lower extremities. The most common complaints are an inability to move the legs and associated severe back and abdominal pain. Abrasions and contusions, with or without focal hematomas, are

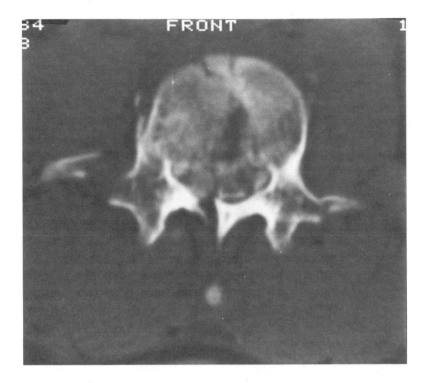

Figure 7. *Computerized tomographic scan of L1 after a severe flexion-rotation injury in a 14-year-old boy. Note that the spinal canal is almost completely obliterated by bony fragments.*

commonly present over the back and aid in determining the mechanism of injury. With severe compression, a widening of the interspinous distance can be palpated. In such circumstances, scoliosis, kyphosis, or excessive lordosis of the spine may be evident. Fractures of the scapula with associated localized hematomas should alert the physician to the possible presence of a thoracic compression-dislocation fracture; with such an injury a significant rotational force may have been applied to the spine. Except in the case of rib fractures, only rarely are other major injuries associated with thoracic spinal fractures.[15,16]

Instability of the thoracic or thoracolumbar spine after injury depends on the degree of damage to posterior elements. If the bony and ligamentous posterior structures remain intact, the fracture is most likely stable. When fracture of the articular processes (facet joints) is present or rupture of the posterior ligaments is suspected, the injury is potentially unstable. A fracture is definitely unstable if the posterior elements are completely disrupted and vertebral body displacement or dislocation is present by radiographic examination. With simple hyperflexion thoracic wedge fractures, the only treatment necessary is simple bed rest, as such fractures are asymptomatic within a few weeks. If the degree of vertebral compression is greater than 25 percent or severe back or abdominal pain or associated injuries are present, hospitalization is indicated. Reduction of wedge fractures by traction or operative methods is not indicated since these methods make no significant difference in the end result. External support in the form of braces is generally not needed unless for symptomatic purposes. Activity can be initiated rapidly and gradually increased depending upon the patient's symptoms and tolerance.

The treatment of more severe degrees of thoracic compression fracture should consist of bed rest until pain relief is achieved. A plaster or molded plastic body cast should be used for immobilization while healing is occurring— generally two to three months. The prognosis for full recovery is excellent. Even with severe compression fractures, spinal fusion is rarely necessary in this region in the child. However, follow-up through skeletal spinal maturity is necessary to watch for the delayed development of scoliosis or kyphosis secondary to endplate damage.

Unstable thoracic fractures, with or without associated neurologic deficits, will require early spinal fusion. Complete bed rest, with or without the use of pelvic traction, is indicated until fusion is performed. Unstable fractures will result in a rapidly progressive spinal deformity with the potential for further neurologic compromise if fusion is not performed.

Repeated radiographs following compression fractures of the immature spine may show a restoration of vertebral body height. The younger the child and the less severe the compression, the greater the chances are for complete restoration of vertebral body height with growth and development. Children with severe fractures or children over ten years of age will usually show some permanent asymmetrical wedging of the vertebral bodies.

LUMBAR FRACTURES

The lumbar spine rarely is injured severely in children. Flexion and distraction injuries are the most common type of injuries in this region. Flexion injuries produce mild to moderate wedge fractures of the vertebral bodies. Generally, in children, the vertebral body wedges and gives way before the posterior longitudinal ligament ruptures and the posterior elements are involved. Thus, such injuries are rarely associated with neurologic deficits. However, if the flexion force is severe, a bursting fracture of the vertebral body may occur with the potential for significant compromise of the neural canal.

Distraction injuries are the most severe lumbar spinal injuries and may be associated with lap seat belts. Such injuries occur most frequently at the L1 to L3 levels and result from sudden deceleration in the presence of a restraint, such as a seat belt. This deceleration force shears the discs and dislocates the facets. The superior facets of the lower vertebra dislocate anterior to the inferior facets of the upper vertebra. The history and physical examination in this type of injury is very similar to that in those patients with flexion-rotation injuries of the thoracic spine. Frequently abdominal contusions secondary to the lap belt may be present. Severe neurologic deficits are usually present.[2]

Isolated fractures involving the neural arch, facet, transverse, or spinous processes account for the remainder of the lumbar spinal injuries. The most common mechanism of such injuries is a direct blow. Anterior body wedge fractures, facet fractures, and neural arch fractures are best treated with external support until evidence of healing is obtained by clinical and radiographic evaluation. Fractures of the transverse process or spinous process require only symptomatic treatment. External support or bracing may or may not be used depending on the child's discomfort with activity.

Stable wedge fractures of the lumbar spine without associated neurologic deficit are best treated with external support such as a plaster body cast or a molded plastic body cast. However, in such a situation, careful radiological and neurologic follow-up should be undertaken. Most fractures will become stable after 12 weeks of immobilization. The development of paravertebral callus is a sign of healing that can be followed radiographically. When such fractures occur in prepubertal children, some advocate continued bracing until the majority of spinal growth has ceased (age 14 in girls, age 16 in boys) to prevent any spinal deformity from developing. Once the external support is removed, flexion-extension films should be obtained to ensure that stable healing has occurred.

If the posterior elements are fractured in combination with the vertebral body or any subluxation is present, then postural reduction is the best method of initial treatment. Various traction devices are available to provide controlled reduction and immediate stabilization.

If operative treatment is indicated because of gross spinal instability or significant neural canal compromise with associated neurologic disability or conservative therapy fails because of instability or progressive spinal deformity, operative fusion is required. The surgical procedure selected (anterior, posterior, or combined) as well as the type of internal fixation utilized is best determined on an individual basis, depending on the mechanism of the injury and the bony abnormalities present.

Unstable injuries, such as distraction injuries and, usually, burst compression fractures, will require fusion. The use of either bone graft, plates, compression or distraction rods, or some combination of these methods depends on many factors. If no neurologic impairment is associated with such injuries and only closed reduction is used for treatment, then progressive deformity, pain, and/or neurologic deficit may occur. If significant neurologic deficit is present and complete from the time of injury, then open operation is indicated for the purposes of stabilization. If a partial conus injury or cauda equina injury is present, then early operation is indicated not only for stabilization but for removal of any compressive elements within the neural canal. Postoperatively, external stabilization with a spica or body cast is required for two to three months. As with those injuries treated nonoperatively, careful radiological follow-up on a long-term basis is essential to be aware of progressive scoliosis, excessive lordosis, or kyphosis.

SPINAL CORD INJURY WITHOUT RADIOGRAPHIC ABNORMALITIES

The entity of spinal cord injury without radiographic abnormality (SCIWORA) has been noted to occur not infrequently in children. The anatomical and biomechanical characteristics of the infantile spine predispose it to subluxations and other types of injuries that may spontaneously reduce, leaving little or no radiographic evidence of abnormality, while at the same time resulting in severe degrees of neurologic compromise secondary to cord injury.[1,13] The incidence of SCIWORA varies from a low of 2 percent of all spinal cord injuries seen in children to a high of 50 percent of all spinal cord injuries seen in children under the age of 15.[3,4,20] While the occurrence of spinal cord injury without radiographic abnormality is seen in adults, the most common type of neurologic lesion is that of the central cord syndrome, which occurs secondary to a hyperextension in-

jury in patients that have spondylitic disease of the cervical
spine. In children, however, the neurologic lesions associated with SCIWORA tend to be much more severe.[4,14]

There appears to be a significant difference in the
neurologic status of children less than eight years of age and
those over eight years of age with SCIWORA. Neurologic
injuries encountered in children younger than eight years of
age tend to be much more serious than those seen in older
children. More of the recorded complete cord transections
and the more severe incomplete lesions have been found in
children under eight years of age. When SCIWORA occurs
in older children, the lesions tend to be milder with a better
prognosis.[14]

It has also been noted that a large proportion of children suffering from SCIWORA will have a late onset of
neurologic symptoms. In the cases reported by Pang and
Wilberger, 52 percent of the children had delayed onset of
paralysis.[13] Concomitantly, many of these children recalled
initial transient symptoms, including paresthesia, numbness, or a subjective feeling of paralysis. These initial
symptoms resolved and the delayed onset of neurologic deficits occurred anywhere from 2 to 24 hours later. The exact
mechanism of this delayed onset of neurologic lesions is
unknown. It may be related to the well-known ligamentous
laxity in children, which is further compromised by injury
resulting in insipient instability. Repeated movement over
several hours may result in delayed cord injury. Also, a
vascular mechanism may result in delayed paralysis.

As the diagnosis of this entity requires careful radiological investigation, flexion-extension films are often obtained. If immediate instability is evident by the flexion-
extension study, cervical fusion or halo fixation is recommended. If no abnormalities are demonstrated, especially in
the presence of significant spinal cord injury, then a complete radiological workup including tomograms, CT scan,
myelograms, and possibly magnetic resonance scanning is
indicated.

VASCULAR INJURIES SECONDARY
TO SPINAL TRAUMA

Since 1952, when attention was first drawn to the possibility of vertebral or carotid artery trauma secondary to cervical spine injuries, a large number of cases have been reported. The carotid artery can be damaged by the rotational or torsional forces associated with the spinal injury. Occasionally, the carotid may be compressed against the lower cervical or upper thoracic vertebral bodies. Another potential site for carotid injury is at the point where the internal carotid artery passes around the carotid tubercle at the level of C1. The vertebral artery is even more susceptible to injury in association with cervical spinal injuries because of its anatomical relationship to bone. Shortly after it arises from the subclavian or aortic arch the vertebral artery enters the foramina transversaria of C6 and ascends through this bony canal up to C1 where it crosses a groove in the lamina of the atlas under the occipital condyles and subsequently into the foramen magnum (Fig. 8). As such, the vertebral artery is tethered to the cervical spine and is subject to shearing forces when excessive rotation, extension, or flexion occur. Similarly, the artery may be compressed under the occipital condyles when flexion or extension occurs at this level. Many studies have shown that flow in both the vertebral and carotid vessels may be significantly reduced by neck movements well within the physiological range.

Injuries to the vertebral or carotid arteries may take the form of immediate occlusion, delayed thrombosis, spasm, intimal tears with dissection, traumatic aneurysms, or arteriovenous fistula formation. As such, the clinical manifestations of the injury may be immediate or delayed in onset. Similarly, the resultant neurologic deficits may be transient or permanent. In the case of vertebral artery injuries, immediate death may result secondary to brain stem ischemia if there is insufficient collateral blood flow.

The possibility of vascular injury must always be borne

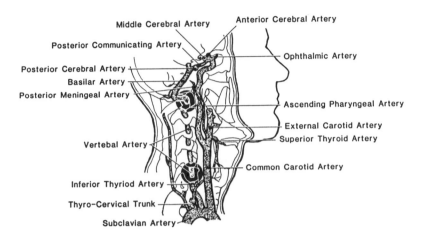

Figure 8. Schematic representation of the relationship of carotid and vertebral arteries to the cervical spine. The dark circles indicate the regions of the vertebral artery most susceptible to injury.

in mind when dealing with cervical spinal injuries. In the presence of neurologic deficit that cannot be explained adequately on the basis of the bony injury to the spine, angiography should be considered to evaluate the carotid and vertebral vessels. With any delayed neurologic deficit, even in the presence of significant bony injury, carotid or vertebral injury should be suspected and angiography considered. Depending on the nature of the vascular injury and the associated neurologic condition, various treatments can be instituted. Direct surgical exploration may be indicated in cases of acute, immediate, carotid, or vertebral occlusion. Anticoagulation may be indicated for delayed thrombosis or intimal tears with dissection. Surgical reconstruction is necessary when traumatic aneurysms develop.

REFERENCES

1. Ahmann PA, Smith SA, Schwartz JF, et al: Spinal cord infarction due to minor trauma in children. Neurology 25:301–307, 1975.
2. Burke DC, Murray DD: The management of thoracic and thoracal

lumbar injuries of the spine with neurological involvement. *J Bone Jt Surg (Br)* 58:72–78, 1976.

3. Chèshire DJE: The pediatric syndrome of traumatic myelopathy without demonstrable vertebral injury. *Paraplegia* 15:74–85, 1977.
4. Evans DK: Anterior cervical subluxation. *J Bone Jt Surg (Br)* 58B:318–321, 1976.
5. Ewald FC: Fracture of the odontoid process in a 17-month old infant treated with a halo. *J Bone Jt Surg* 53A:1636–1640, 1971.
6. Fielding JW, Hawkins RJ: Atlanto axial rotary fixation. *J Bone Jt Surg* 59A:37–45, 1977.
7. Gaufin LM, Goodman SJ: Cervical spine injuries in children. Problems in management. *J Bone Jt Surg* 42:179–184, 1975.
8. Gilles FH, Bina M, Sotrel A: Infantile atlanto occipital instability. *Am J Dis in Child* 133:30–37, 1979.
9. Griffiths SC: Fracture of the odontoid process in children. *J Pediatr Surg* 7:680,1972.
10. Marlin AE, Williams GR, Lee JF: Jefferson fractures in children. *J Neurosurg* 58:277–279, 1983.
11. Murphy MJ, Ogden JA, Southwick WO: Spinal stabilization in acute spine injuries. *Surg Clinic of North America* 60:1035, 1980.
12. Pang D, Wilberger JE: Spinal cord injury without radiographic abnormalities in children. *J Neurosurg* 57:114–129, 1982.
13. Pang D, Wilberger JE: Traumatic atlanto occipital dislocation with survival. Case Report in a Review. *Neurosurg* 5:503–508, 1980.
14. Papavasiliou V: Traumatic subluxation of the cervical spine during childhood. *Orthop Clinics of North America* 9:945–955, 1978.
15. Rolander SD, Blair WE: Deformation and fracture to the lumbar vertebral end plate. *Orthop Clinics of North America* 6:75, 1975.
16. Rucksthuhl J, Morscher E, Jani L: Behandlung und prognose von wirhelfrakturen im kindes—und jugendalter. *Chirurg* 47:458, 1976.
17. Seimon LP: Fracture of the odontoid process in young children. *J Bone Jt Surg* 59A:943–948, 1977.
18. Sherk HH, Nickelson JT, Chung SMK: Fractures of the odontoid process in young children. *J Bone Jt Surg (Br)* 60A:921, 1978.
19. Sherk HH, Schut L, Lane JM: Fractures and dislocation of the cervical spine in children. *Orthop Clinics of North America* 7:593–604, 1976.
20. Taylor AR: The mechanism of injury to the spinal cord in the neck without damage to the vertebral column. *J Bone Jt Surg (Br)* 33:543–547, 1951.
21. Taylor AR, Blackwood W: Paraplegia in hyperextension injuries with normal radiographic appearances. *J Bone Jt. Surg (Br)* 30:245–248, 1948.
22. Weiss MH, Kaufman B: Hangman's fracture in an infant. *Am J Dis in Child* 126:268–269, 1973.

Chapter 5

ACUTE CARE OF THE SPINAL CORD INJURED CHILD

Once the immediate problems of the spinal cord injured child have been managed, attention must be directed toward preventing the many complications that may occur acutely following spinal cord injury. The first week to ten days following a spinal cord injury are the most important as the majority of life-threatening complications occur during this time. Special attention must be directed toward preventing and treating any complications that may occur as a result of pulmonary, cardiovascular, urinary tract, or gastrointestinal problems related to the spinal cord injury. Similarly, careful and early attention must be given to skin care as well as to nutrition of the spinal cord injured child.

PULMONARY COMPLICATIONS

Pulmonary complications are the single most common cause of morbidity and mortality acutely following spinal cord injury. Chest complications are the result of impaired normal breathing mechanisms secondary to diaphragmatic, intercostal, respiratory, and abdominal muscle paralysis, while associated injuries such as chest trauma, rib fractures, or head injury will further increase the risk of significant pulmonary complications.[18,22] The higher the spinal cord injury, the greater the incidence of pulmonary problems;

however, complications can occur even in conus level lesions. Atelectasis and subsequent bronchial pneumonia are common in spinal cord injured children. While pulmonary embolism is a major complication in adult spinal cord injury, this is seen rarely in children. Paralysis of the respiratory muscles makes deep breathing and coughing extremely difficult. As deep breathing and coughing are the two primary protective mechanisms in the normal child, this paralysis predisposes to the retention of secretions and increases the risk for atelectasis and pneumonia. Similarly, abdominal muscular weakness prevents effective coughing to clear secretions. Use of skeletal traction requires keeping the child in a recumbent position, which further complicates pulmonary care. The recumbent position allows for pooling of secretions in the dependent regions of the lungs and also increases the likelihood of aspiration.

With high level spinal cord injury and associated acute respiratory insufficiency, oral or nasotracheal intubation is most likely performed during the initial acute resuscitation and treatment. In the presence of a cervical cord injury, if the child is not already intubated, careful observation must be maintained to ensure that insidious respiratory insufficiency does not develop. Arterial blood gas studies and measurements of vital capacity should be performed at regular intervals, and agitation, restlessness, or disorientation should be clinically watched as signs of insufficient oxygenation. Some physicians advocate endotracheal intubation and mechanical ventilation for hypoventilation, irregular breathing, or unexplained air hunger even if arterial blood gases are normal.[22]

There are several indications for the use of mechanical ventilation in children with spinal cord injuries:

1. Complete respiratory insufficiency secondary to a high level cervical injury with no diaphragmatic, intercostal, abdominal, or accessory respiratory muscle function;

2. Partial respiratory insufficiency secondary to a high cervical cord injury;
3. Respiratory insufficiency associated with spinal cord injury but occurring secondary to broncho-pneumonia, aspiration, or severe abdominal distention;
4. The presence of associated chest injuries, such as multiple rib fractures or pulmonary contusions.

Some authors feel that almost every child with a significant cervical spinal cord injury will require ventilatory assistance at some point during the acute stage of their injury. An endotracheal tube with a soft cuff can be safely left in place for up to 10 to 14 days. Unless there is a high cervical cord injury above the C3 level, the vast majority of children will be weaned from the respirator during this time and will not require a tracheostomy. However, if it appears that the respiratory insufficiency will be longer lasting, or certainly in the presence of a high cord injury in which the chances for recovery of independent respiratory function are small, then a tracheostomy should be performed sooner than the 10- to 14-day time period.

Another potential complication of high cervical injuries is that of sleep apnea. From anatomical studies, it is known that automatic respiration is regulated by the reticulospinal system that lies in the anterior lateral column of the spinal cord from C1 to C3. If these pathways are damaged significantly then only voluntary respiration, which is dependent upon consciousness, is possible, and cessation of breathing may occur during sleep. This syndrome should be carefully watched for in children with high level cervical spinal cord injuries and requires the use of an apnea monitor on a continuous basis for the first week to ten days following injury.

Constant vigilance must be maintained in order to rapidly diagnose and treat the complication of pneumonia should it occur. Repeated chest x-ray films are the most reliable and effective means of rapid diagnosis of this complication. Children who are receiving ventilatory support should have chest x-ray films performed on a daily or every-other-day basis. Children with tracheostomies in place should have a routine chest x-ray film weekly during their acute hospital stay. Similarly, a chest x-ray film should be performed if symptoms develop such as cough, chest discomfort, or apnea. Development of tachycardia, tachypnea, or fever should alert the physician to the possibility of pneumonia. Use of prophylactic antibiotics is not encouraged, even in those children who require prolonged intubation or tracheostomy. The routine use of prophylactic antibiotics significantly increases in the incidence of serious antibiotic-resistant pulmonary infections. Although pathogenic organisms commonly are found in routine tracheal cultures in such children, they most often represent bacterial colonization and not infection. If clinical evidence of pulmonary infection does develop, then it should be treated vigorously with appropriate antibiotics based on sensitivity studies from sputum and blood cultures.

CARDIOVASCULAR CARE

Aside from vasogenic spinal shock, which has been dealt with separately, several other complications associated with the cardiovascular system may be encountered in the spinal cord injured child and require special attention.[13]

Orthostatic hypotension readily occurs when a quadriplegic or paraplegic is raised from the horizontal to the vertical position. The drop in blood pressure may be so precipitous and severe as to result in syncope. Several cases of severe bradycardia and subsequent cardiac arrest have been reported. Orthostatic hypotension is the result of a rapid influx of blood into the splanchnic and lower limb vessels that subsequently are unable to return this blood to the heart because of the generalized vasomotor paralysis that is present secondary to the spinal cord injury. Thus, it is important to avoid any rapid change in position in children with high level spinal cord injuries.[10]

Paroxysmal hypertension may occur secondary to a mass sympathetic discharge (also known as a mass reflex). Along with the rise in blood pressure, there may be associated sweating, flushing of the face, nasal congestion, shivering, pilomotor erection, headaches, and tachycardia. If this mass reflex occurs, attention should be focused immediately on the bowel or bladder.[9] When the bowel or bladder become overly distended, afferent reflexes from these organs set off sympathetic outflow from the thoracolumbar cord. If the child has a cervical spinal injury, then these reflexes cannot be blocked by descending pathways. At its most severe form, this mass reflex may result in changes in levels of consciousness, seizures, and apnea. Treatment should be directed toward the stimulus that first initiated the mass reflex. Bladder distension can be corrected by unblocking an indwelling Foley catheter or by catheterization. Bowel distension is most often secondary to rectal distension from impactions that can be relieved by enemas or other similar measures.[3]

Bradycardia is not infrequently seen in association with cervical spinal cord injuries. In the first seven to ten days following injury, the bradycardia may be so pronounced as to produce hypotension and syncope. The bradycardia results from loss of sympathetic outflow to the heart with subsequent vagal hyperactivity. The bradycardia, if symptomatic, can be reversed with atropine. All children with cervical spinal cord injuries should be monitored electrocardiographically on a continuous basis for the first week following the injury to watch for this complication.

Thermoregulatory dysfunction is another manifestation of the lack of vascular control secondary to spinal cord injury. With lesions above the C8 level, the child essentially becomes poikilothermic. The child is unable to vasodilate or vasoconstrict and, therefore, unable to retain or dissipate heat in response to the outside temperature. Thus, if the outside temperature drops, body core temperature will drop as well. With rising temperatures, body temperature will increase. Care must be taken, using appropriate cooling or warming techniques, to prevent the body temperature from fluctuating excessively.[19]

GASTROINTESTINAL CARE

Paralytic ileus, a manifestation of generalized autonomic dysfunction, occurs almost universally in children with cervical and thoracic spinal cord injuries. The development of a paralytic ileus with subsequent abdominal distension can be harmful from several standpoints: 1) progressive abdominal distension can result in respiratory compromise by elevating the diaphragm and compressing the lung parenchyma; 2) progressive gastric distension can result in vomiting with the subsequent risk for pulmonary aspiration; 3) bowel distension may set off the undesirable mass autonomic reflexes previously described. As the paralytic ileus can neither be prevented nor directly treated, the primary treatment should consist of placement of a nasogastric tube to maintain constant aspiration of gastric contents. This will effectively prevent progressive abdominal distension and its associated complications. The nasogastric tube should be left in place until spinal shock subsides and peristaltic function returns as evidenced by the return of active bowel sounds or the passage of flatus or stool.

Once the problem of paralytic ileus resolves, bowel retraining and regulation must be initiated and maintained to prevent severe constipation, impaction, and associated undesirable side effects. A bowel regimen should be initiated during the acute hospital phase to provide for a daily bowel movement. The most effective bowel regimens to establish a daily routine make use of a combination of rectal suppositories, enemas, and oral purgatives.

More severe and life-threatening abdominal complications on an acute basis, such as splenic rupture or liver lacerations, or on a chronic basis, such as bowel obstruction, bowel perforation, appendicitis, or other similar conditions, may be obscured because of a relative lack of pain perception in children with spinal cord injury.[5] Occasionally, vague pain may be appreciated secondary to autonomic visceral afferents that are conducted into the spinal cord via the splanchnic, hypogastric, or pelvic nerves. Also, if the spinal cord lesion is not above the C5 level, referred pain secondary to diaphragmatic irritation may be felt in the shoulder region. Other signs of ongoing abdominal complications, such as temperature elevation, elevated white blood cell count, or associated ileus are not reliable signs for the identification of abdominal disease in such patients. Similarly, clinical examination may be misleading as localized abdominal tenderness, muscle guarding, and rigidity may be absent even in the presence of severe peritonitis. Thus, it must be recognized that children with spinal cord injuries can develop such abdominal complications and one must watch carefully for any indirect signs that may point to an ongoing abdominal problem. Use of the CT scan and sonography may prove extremely useful in evaluating possible abdominal complications.[4,15]

GENITOURINARY TRACT CARE

The main source of systemic infection in acutely spinal cord injured children is the bladder. The bladder also can account for significant long-term disability secondary to associated renal damage if appropriate care is not undertaken early on following the spinal cord injury. The somatic musculature of the bladder is flaccid during spinal shock, although the bladder itself is not completely atonic because of a rich intramural autonomic network. Thus, during spinal shock, spontaneous voiding occurs only when the bladder overflows. In children, reflex micturition usually returns within a few days. The micturition center is located in the second, third, and fourth sacral segments and is linked to the detrusor muscle of the bladder by the corresponding nerve roots. Normally, the spinal reflex center is dominated by higher medullary and cortical centers that control micturition. When there is complete injury to the spinal cord above this center, it is cut off from all higher control; as soon as the phase of spinal shock has passed, micturition may start automatically on a reflex basis. At this point the bladder is comparable to that of a newborn child and is variously termed an automatic bladder or an upper motor neuron bladder. If the spinal cord injury is in the lower lumbar or sacral regions, the sacral reflex center and/or the nerve roots supplying the bladder may be destroyed and subsequently the bladder will be devoid of any spinal reflex control. Such a situation is known as an autonomous or lower neuron bladder.[7,10]

The use of indwelling Foley catheters in the acute spinal cord injured child has all but been abandoned except in cases of multiple associated injuries with or without associated shock. In these cases, urine output must be monitored carefully on an hourly basis. It is well known that infection will occur within 48 to 96 hours of the placement of an indwelling Foley catheter. One study found that within 96 hours of indwelling catheter placement, 98 percent of patients developed bacteremia despite the use of prophylactic antibiotics. Aside from the acute problem of infection, the long-term use of indwelling Foley catheters may be associated with significant urethral, bladder, and renal complications.[16,17]

Intermittent catheterization using sterile techniques is the recommended treatment for control of bladder distension after acute spinal cord injury. Initially, the child should be catheterized every three to four hours until urine is passed either voluntarily or automatically. If the catheterizations yield more than 300 to 400 cc, this indicates that the bladder is being overdistended and that the time interval between catheterizations should be shortened accordingly.[14] The use of prophylactic antibiotics when performing intermittent catheterizations are not indicated and specific urinary tract infections should be treated with appropriate antibiotics. If the catheterizations are going to be carried out for a prolonged period of time or other complicating factors are present, then urinary antiseptics, such as Mandelamine or nitrofurantoin, may be used to aid in maintaining urinary sterility.[6,8,17]

Bladder reeducation should begin promptly in the acute hospital phase. In the case of the automatic bladder, the reflex arc is intact and reeducation consists of evoking the automatic action of the bladder by reflex. With the autonomous bladder, absence of the reflex arc excludes any automatic functioning, and the child must either rely on contracting the abdominal muscles or exerting external pressure with the hands to effect bladder emptying. Various drugs also have been found to be useful in establishing automatic function of the upper motor neuron bladder. Bethanechol chloride, a cholinergic agonist, may be quite effective for hypoactivity of the detrusor muscle. Phenoxybenzamine has been found to be useful for associated spasticity or hypertonicity of the internal urethral sphincter.

SKIN CARE

Development of decubitus or pressure ulcerations are an unacceptable complication of spinal cord injury in children. Immobility and the lack of sensation predispose to pressure necrosis of the skin and subsequent skin breakdown. Prolonged pressure over the skin, particularly over bony prominences, must be avoided. In the acute stages of

spinal cord injury during the early weeks of immobilization, pressure points to the skin can be avoided only by
turning the child every two hours. Currently available apparatuses such as the Stryker frame and Roto-rest beds
allow for controlled movement of the child without com-
promising spinal stability. Water mattresses and alternating
air mattresses prevent an excessive buildup of pressure at
any one point on the skin. Daily examinations should be
made of the most vulnerable parts of the body for the development of pressure ulceration. In small children, the
back of the head is particularly vulnerable to the development of a pressure ulceration. In older children, the most
common sites are over the posterior iliac crests and spine. If
plaster immobilization must be used, such as the Minerva
jacket or a plaster halo vest, extreme care must be taken to
prevent skin breakdown at the sites of pressure from the
casts. This can be accomplished by generous padding with
lamb's wool, foam, or other similar substances.

Once skin breakdown does occur, it is often extremely
difficult to treat because of the lack of innervation to the
skin and the poor vascular control, both have a significant
adverse effect on healing.[18]

NUTRITIONAL CARE

Severe injury to the spinal cord, similar to other systemic insults and injuries, produces an immediate, often
sustained, catabolic response. The benefits of careful and
early attention to nutritional status have been repeatedly
shown. Children have a limited ability to tolerate prolonged
periods of catabolism because of their intrinsically high
basal metabolic rates and their small caloric reserves. The
child initially will respond to catabolism by breaking down
available protein stores to provide substrates for gluconeo-
genesis. The new glucose that is produced supplies obligat-
ory needs of the central nervous system for glucose as an

energy substrate. However, the breakdown of protein cannot continue indefinitely as the protein reserves of the body available for energy substrate are normally in the form of functioning enzymes, cellular building blocks, and muscles. Continued protein catabolism, therefore, represents a loss of essential biologic components. Starvation-related mortality results when one-third to one-half of the body protein has been lost. At this low level of protein reserve, the general repair functions of the body are affected adversely by severe muscle wasting, ineffective coughing, pneumonia, impaired wound healing, poor resistance to infection, and diminished synthesis of enzymes and plasma proteins.[12,21]

If the GI tract is functional, it is by far the best means of supplying protein and calories. Use of a flexible, small bore pediatric feeding tube prevents the possible complications of gastric irritation, gastroesophageal reflux, and aspiration. Various commercial products are available for enteral hyperalimentation. If a routine form cannot be utilized because of intestinal malabsorption, elemental formulas are available containing amino acids, triglycerides, and simple sugars. Occasionally, if the GI tract is not functional or significant associated injuries prevent its use, total parenteral nutrition may need to be instituted. Total parenteral nutrition provides all essential nutrients intravenously using a 25 percent dextrose and a 3 percent to 5 percent amino-acid solution. Careful attention must be paid to the details of total parenteral nutrition administration so as to prevent many of the metabolic and central venous catheter-associated complications that can occur if this therapeutic modality is utilized in a haphazard manner.[11,12]

It is extremely important that proper nutrition be supplied early to children with severe spinal cord injuries as protein catabolism begins several hours after the injury and continues throughout the period of relative starvation that follows. Complications during convalescence will worsen the protein breakdown process. Any attempts to reduce

protein wasting and to provide adequate calories to coun-
teract infection and stress and, ultimately, to induce tissue
anabolism for wound repair must be instituted vigorously at
the earliest possible opportunity. Early consideration of the
total nutritional needs of the child with spinal cord injury
can be translated into effective, supportive, and preventive
therapy using a wide range of interventions. Nutritional
support, when indicated, should be instituted early. Maintenance of good nutritional status is preferable to the rehabilitation of the malnourished infant or child since it is
easier, less risky, less expensive, and optimizes the chances
for recovery.[1,24]

Children with spinal cord injuries may also develop
significant electrolyte imbalances. Profound hyponatremia
may develop as a result of the syndrome of inappropriate
antidiuretic hormone secretion (SIADH). The SIADH can
occur with any insult to the nervous system and results in
hyponatremia, excessive renal excretion of sodium, and
hyperosmolar urine in the face of serum hypoosmolarity.
Serum sodium drops too low and seizures may result.
SIADH is corrected generally by fluid restriction until the
hyponatremia is reversed. If fluid restriction is ineffective,
or if the degree and duration of fluid restriction has significant adverse effects on the nutritional status of the child,
consideration should be given to other modalities of treatment. If very low serum sodiums associated with seizures
occur, more aggressive therapy is indicated. The use of loop
diuretics in association with the replacement of fluid losses
with 3 percent saline solution has proved to be extremely
effective in rapidly returning serum sodium to normal in
the face of SIADH.[2,20]

Severe hyperkalemia can occur in children with spinal
cord injury and associated quadriplegia and paraplegia
after the administration of succinylcholine.[23] Elevation in
serum potassium may be so severe as to result in ventricular
fibrillation. Succinylcholine is a depolarizing agent used in
anesthesia. The clinical explanation for the sudden rise in

serum potassium levels is that denervated muscle responds atypically to depolarization thus releasing excessive potassium from the cell membrane. It has been strongly recommended that this agent not be used for any child with a severe spinal cord injury up to 90 days after the injury.

REFERENCES

1. Ballinger WS (ed): *Manual of Surgical Nutrition.* Philadelphia, W.T. Saunders, 1975, pp 46–50, 122–162.
2. Bartter FC, Schwartz WB: The syndrome of inappropriate secretion of anti-diuretic hormone. *Am J Med* 42:793–796, 1967.
3. Bors E, French JD: Management of paroxysmal hypertension following injuries to cervical and upper thoracic segments of the spinal cord. *Arch Surg* 64:803–812, 1952.
4. Charney KJ, Juler GL, Comarr AE: General surgery problems in patients with spinal cord injuries. *Arch Surg* 110:1083–1088, 1975.
5. Cohen TI, Cooper IS: Acute abdominal emergencies in paraplegics. *Am J Surg* 75:19–24, 1948.
6. Comarr AE: Intermittent catheterization for the traumatic cord bladder patient. *J Urol* 108:79–81, 1972.
7. Gibbon NOK: Neurogenic bladder in spinal cord injury. *Neurol Clin N America* 1:147–154, 1974.
8. Guttmann L, Frankel H: The value of intermittent catheterization in the management of traumatic paraplegia and tetraplegia. *Paraplegia* 4:63–84, 1966.
9. Guttmann L, Whitteridge D: Effect of bladder distension on autonomic mechanisms after spinal cord injuries. *Brain* 70:361, 1947.
10. Head H, Riddoch G: Automatic bladder, excessive sweating and some other reflex conditions in gross injuries to spinal cord. *Brain* 40:188–263, 1917.
11. Heird WC, Driscoll JM, Schullinger JN, et al: Intravenous alimentation in pediatric patients. *J Pediatr* 80:351–372, 1972.
12. Irvin TT: Effects of malnutrition and hyperalimentation on wound healing. *Surg, Gynecol Obstet* 146:33–37, 1978.
13. Meincke FW: Regulation of the cardiovascular system in patients with fresh injuries to the spinal cord. *Paraplegia* 9:109–112, 1971.
14. O'Flynn JD: Early management of neuropathic bladder in spinal cord injuries. *Paraplegia* 12:83–86, 1974.
15. O'Hare JM: The acute abdomen in spinal injury patients. *Proc Journals Clin Spinal Injury Conf* 15:113–117, 1966.
16. Owen SE, Finch ET: Bacteriological study of urine from paraplegic patients. *J Neurol* 61:258–264, 1949.
17. Pearman JW: Prevention of urinary tract infection following spinal cord injury. *Paraplegia* 9:95–104, 1971.

18. Pearman JW, England EJ: *The Neurological Management of the Patient Following Spinal Cord Injury.* Springfield IL, Charles C. Thomas, 1973, pp 243–251.
19. Pollack LJ, Boshes B, Chor H, et al: Defects in regulatory mechanisms in autonomic functions in injuries to spinal cord. *J Neurophysiol* 14:85, 1951.
20. Schucart WA, Carroll HJ: Fluid and electrolyte problems in neurosurgical patients. *Contemp Neurosurg* 3, No. 9:1–8, 1983.
21. Scrimshaw NS, Taylor CE, Gordon JE: Interactions of nutrition and infection. *Monogr 57*, World Health Organization, Geneva, Switzerland, 1968.
22. Silver JR: Chest injuries and complications in the early stages of spinal cord injury. *Paraplegia* 5:226–245, 1968.
23. Stone WA, Beech TP, Hamelberg W: Succinylcholine induced hyperkalemia in dogs with transected siatic nerves and spinal cords. *Anesthesiology* 32:515–520, 1970.
24. Winters RW: Total parenteral nutrition in pediatrics. *Pediatrics* 56:17–23, 1975.

Chapter 6

PHARMACOTHERAPY OF SPINAL CORD INJURY

*Frank T. Vertosick Jr. and
James E. Wilberger, Jr.*

Although physiologically fragile, the spinal cord is anatomically quite tough and is rarely lacerated during fracture dislocations of the spine. The vast majority of paralyzing spinal cord injuries (SCI) are the result of spinal cord contusion, not transection. Unfortunately, the unique pathophysiological response of the spinal cord to contusion renders its initial and anatomical preservation during spinal cord injuries clinically meaningless. Even if the cord is anatomically intact following major impact injury, complete dissolution of the injured cord segment usually follows within 48 hours.

It has long been hoped that some way of pharmacologically inhibiting the spinal cord's inherently self-destructive response to impact injury could be found because most clinical SCI spare the continuity of the cord, at least for several hours after injury. The prevention of the pathologic cascade triggered within the wounded spinal cord would hold much promise for enhancing the motor recovery in these tragic cases.

Unfortunately, a successful method of preventing delayed cord necrosis in the clinical setting has not been

111

found even though there has been progress in animal models. Occasionally, an enthusiastic report of a drug's success in enhancing recovery in animals will be presented in the general medical journals or the lay press generating false hope in the patients afflicted with SCI. To deal with the situation adequately, it is important to be aware of the developments in this rapidly changing field. Adequate treatment of the injured spinal cord should attempt to reconcile the pathophysiological events seen after trauma and the possible effects of specific medical or pharmacologic therapy in resolving or arresting the impending pathologic sequence.

THE PATHOPHYSIOLOGICAL RESPONSE TO SPINAL CORD INJURY

For up to several minutes following severe impact injury to the spinal cord, the cord may look grossly and histologically normal. Detailed animal studies of impact SCI, however, have delineated the sequence of pathologic events that transform this normal appearance into an appearance of total focal necrosis and inflammation within 24 to 48 hours of injury (Fig. 1).

Light microscopy shows petechial hemorrhages in the central cord gray matter within 30 minutes of injury. Initially confined to the areas in the anterior horns and about the central canal, these hemorrhages coalesce over several hours and extend into the posterior gray matter and white matter. Two hours after injury, an invasion of microglia and polymorphonuclear leukocytes begins. Nearly half the cord's cross-sectional area is necrotic by the fourth hour after injury. If the initial impact is severe, the entire cross-sectional area of the cord will become necrotic within 48 hours of impact injury. Occasionally, a small rim of white matter may remain. Weeks after injury, only a contracted scar consisting of astrocytes, fibroblasts, and collagen will remain.

In addition to cellular changes, significant vascular changes occur following cord injury. Within two hours of injury there is a significant reduction in spinal cord blood flow. Severe vascular congestion develops and leads to central extravasation of red cells and edema fluid, causing increased cord swelling, a rise in interstitial tissue pressure, and further reduction of cord perfusion. Oxygen tensions fall at the center of the cord and carbon dioxide tensions rise. Vascular autoreactivity is lost and ischemia and infarction ensue.[9,31]

Several biochemical explanations for the cord ischemia that develops after injury have been suggested. Osterholm,

PATHOPHYSIOLOGIC RESPONSE TO SPINAL CORD INJURY

TIME	ANATOMICAL	PHYSIOLOGICAL	BIOCHEMICAL
IMMEDIATE	CORD DEFORMATION		
1 MINUTE		LOSS OF EVOKED POTENTIALS	LIPID PEROXIDATION–FREE RADICAL FORMATION
5 MINUTES	AXONAL SWELLING	VASOCONSTRICTION	
15 MINUTES		DECREASED GREY AND WHITE MATTER BLOOD FLOW	INCREASED THROMBOXANE LEVELS
			INCREASED TISSUE NOREPINEPHRINE LEVELS
30 MINUTES	CENTRAL HEMORRHAGES	ISCHEMIA	PROFOUND TISSUE HYPOXIA
1 HOUR			
4 HOURS	BLOOD VESSEL NECROSIS		
	WHITE MATTER EDEMA		
8 HOURS	CENTRAL HEMATOMA FORMATION		
24 HOURS	WHITE MATTER NECROSIS		

Figure 1. *The pathophysiological responses to spinal cord injury are outlined in the above chart, which indicates the anatomical, physiological, and biochemical derangements that occur within the spinal cord after injury.*

for example, implicates norepinephrine released from disrupted nerve terminals as the cause of increased vasospasm within the cord's substance. He has documented that the levels of norepinephrine rise following cord injury and has shown that minute amounts of the substance injected directly into the cord will produce the same histological picture as is seen following impact injury.[30] Other investigators, however, consider increased lipid degradation as the primary culprit. Lipid degeneration, also known as lipid peroxidation, occurs following the disruption of myelin in cellular lipid bilayers. In addition to enhancing the production of toxic-free radicals, which are in themselves harmful to the cellular elements of the cord, lipid peroxidation leads to an imbalance of prostacyclins and thromboxanes within the injured cord. Both of these substances are products of the prostaglandin synthesizing machinery and are made in the vascular endothelial cells. Thromboxanes are potent vasoconstrictors, while prostacyclins are potent vasodilators and a proper balance of the two is required to maintain normal vascular tone. Some authors have suggested that extensive lipid peroxidation causes a selected degradation of prostacyclins as well as an increased synthesis of thromboxane leading to intense vasoconstriction and secondary ischemia. Many of the pharmacologic agents proposed for the treatment of SCI are directed against the ischemic process that occurs within the contused spinal cord. Hyperbaric oxygen has been tried in the hopes that it would increase oxygen delivery to ischemic tissues during the period of intense spinal vascular constriction. Phenoxybenzamine, haloperidol, and alpha-methyltyrosine have been used to block the adrenergic sequelae of increased tissue levels of norepinephrine and dopamine. Glucocorticoids, the most extensively studied of all the pharmacologic agents used in spinal cord injury, have been shown to reduce lipid peroxidation in vitro and may have a role in restoring the balance between thromboxane and prostacyclins after SCI. Dextran, which theoretically improves blood flow by altering the hemorrheology of the microvasculature, has also been found to be of some benefit in improving recovery from experimental spinal injury.[5,8,11,32]

Unfortunately, despite the extensive research into the pathophysiology and pharmacotherapy of SCI in experimental animals, very little systematic research has been carried out in humans with SCI. Consequently, some detailed understanding of animal models of SCI is important in evaluating the various medical or pharmacologic therapies that have been advocated for such injuries.

ANIMAL MODELS OF SCI

Many ways of inducing calibrated SCI in experimental animals have been devised, ranging from the simple sharp transection of the spinal cord to elaborate implanted epidural balloons. The most popular method, however, is the Allen method proposed in 1911 as a way of simulating human fracture dislocation injuries to the spinal cord.[1]

The Allen method employs a vented tube to guide weighted pellets onto the exposed thoracic dura of experimental animals after the pellets have been dropped from a specified height. The resulting impact injury is calibrated in terms of the impacting pellet's weight (in g) multiplied by the height from which it is dropped (in cm). For example, a 40 g weight dropped along the tube from the height of 10 cm would inflict a 400 g cm impact injury to the cord below. The impact area should be specified and in most modern studies is in the range of 10 mm². An impact injury of 500 g per cm and above is considered severe for larger mammals and will cause significant motor paralysis.

Unfortunately, there is considerable individual variation in the response of different animals of the same species to a given impact injury. For example, if ten identical dogs are wounded with a 450 g cm impact injury, then it is possible to be left with five paraplegic dogs, three spastic but ambulatory dogs, and two dogs with no deficits at all. To overcome this variability, it becomes necessary to use a large number of animals and an objective numerical motor recovery score to follow the animals after injury. In this way, quantitative data can be obtained and differences between control and treated animal groups can be compared for statistical significance. One numerical motor scoring system commonly used is the modified Tarlov scale.[33]

Using the Allen injury method and following the animals over weeks and months, investigators have shown an enhancement of motor recovery with a variety of chemical agents. It must be noted, however, that no study has been published claiming an increased motor recovery following pharmacologic treatment in which the impact injury was sufficient to cause permanent and total paralysis in 100 percent of the control animals. In virtually every impact study, there is significant recovery in untreated as well as treated animals. Thus, much of the literature on animal studies deals with models of incomplete spinal cord injury.[29] Unfortunately, complete spinal cord injury is more common clinically and represents the greater therapeutic dilemma. With this background, the evidence for and against the use of individual pharmacologic agents can be reviewed.

PHARMACOLOGIC AGENTS IN SPINAL CORD INJURY

Glucocorticoids

Although many agents have been found to be beneficial in the treatment of experimental spinal injuries, only steroids have achieved common clinical application in this regard. Historically, dexamethasone became the first chemical agent to be rigorously evaluated in an animal model. In 1969, Ducker and Hamit showed an improved motor recovery in beagle dogs when dexamethasone was given intramuscularly following a 375 g/cm impact injury. Results of eleven additional animal trials of either dexamethasone or methylprednisolone have been published since Ducker and Hamit's landmark paper. Eight studies found that steroids significantly enhanced motor recovery in treated animals, two studies found that steroids at least improved the histological appearance of the injured cord (but not the clinical outcome of the cord injury), and one found no benefit to steroid therapy at all. The majority of the data was obtained in dogs or cats subjected to Allen injuries in the range of 375 to 660 g cm of force.[4,9,10]

In addition to the animal trials, a wealth of in vitro evidence has been gathered to justify the use of steroids in human SCI. For example, Hall and Braughler showed that intravenous methylprednisolone inhibits the lipid peroxidation that is triggered within the injured cord of cats following spinal cord injury. A variety of studies have shown that steroids increase the excitability of neurons leading Hall and Braughler to speculate in their excellent review that steroids may help a few axons and neurons that survived to "take up the slack" left behind by the dead cellular elements. The conventional view of steroid action in SCI attributes their potential therapeutic benefit to their known antiedema properties, but careful animal investigation has demonstrated that the improved motor recovery obtained through the use of steroids does not correlate with the reduction of cord edema.[19,20]

If Hall and Braughler are correct, and steroids do act via the inhibition of lipid peroxidation, then clinicians must rethink the time interval between initial injury and initiation of therapy. According to Hall and Braughler, peroxidation starts within minutes of injury and has done irreversible cord injury by one hour postinjury. Thus, if steroids are to be of clinical benefit, they must be given at least within one hour after injury. Unfortunately, this is often impossible in the clinical setting.

Excluding anecdotal reports and nonrandomized series, there has been only one randomized trial of steroids in human SCI. Published in early 1984 by Bracken and colleagues, this was a multicenter double-blind randomized trial of high dose methylprednisolone (1,000 mg bolus followed by 250 mg every 6 hours IV) versus conventional dose methylprednisolone (100 mg bolus followed by 25 mg every 6 hours IV) in patients with complete or incomplete SCI. No patients were denied therapeutic steroids, and therapy with both regimens was continued for ten days after injury. The data of 330 patients were entered between 1979 and 1981. The authors concluded that there was no difference in the sensory or motor recovery of the high dose steroid group versus the conventional dose group, while complications such as mortality and postoperative wound infections were more common in the high dose steroid treatment group. Even though there were no control patients in the study, the overall clinical results of this trial suggest that steroids may not alter the clinical course of SCI.[3] As a result of this trial, a new multicenter trial using steroids versus no steroids in spinal cord injury is presently underway.

There has been considerable concern over the possible side effects of steroid therapy on a routine basis. Conn and Blitzer argued that the risk of gastrointestinal hemorrhage during steroid therapy is probably no greater than it would be in a similar group of highly stressed patients not on steroids. Furthermore, even high dose steroids will not depress the pituitary adrenal axis over a short treatment period (less than ten days) and the risk of wound infection and dehiscence may be enhanced by short-term therapy with steroids but the evidence is inconclusive.[6]

Nevertheless, the high cost of steroid therapy, together with lingering doubts about potential complications have forced clinicians to reevaluate their continued use for human SCI. While the animal evidence is impressive, this literature deals with incomplete cord injuries using impact injuries that are far below those involved in human fracture dislocation injuries. Moreover, the recent in vitro evidence suggests that steroids may only be a benefit if administered within minutes of injury. The final answer to this problem awaits further clinical trials.[7,18,21,26,28]

Catecholamine Blockade (Osterholm Theory)

Osterholm proposed that the decrease in spinal cord blood flow observed following impact injury is secondary to the release of catecholamines (specifically norepinephrine) from the injured neural elements. In his comprehensive review of his catecholamine theory of postinjury spinal cord necrosis, Osterholm outlines three categories of experimental studies to support his theory of postinjury spinal cord ischemia: 1) studies showing that norepinephrine increases after experimental impact injury; 2) studies showing that minute quantities of norepinephrine when injected into the cords of animals will produce lesions identical to the hemorrhagic necrosis seen after impact injuries; 3) studies showing improved motor recovery in animals treated with adrenergic blockade following experimental spinal lesions.[31]

Hendemen et al., however, published data that contradicted Osterholm's theory. These investigators found that the level of norepinephrine declined after a 420 g centiimpact injury in cats while the levels of dopamine rose.[22] Osterholm, on the other hand, argued that dopamine has no role in the pathogenesis of postinjury necrosis citing other studies that document a fall in postinjury dopamine level. Moreover, as Osterholm points out in his review, there are no documented dopamine receptors in the mammalian spinal cord. The question as to whether the norepinephrine levels rise or fall after spinal cord trauma remains unresolved. However, even if the norepinephrine levels were to rise following injury, this is not evidence that the substance is a causative factor in SCI any more than the rise in serum creatinine phosphokinase levels that often follow myocardial infarction is evidence that creatinine phosphokinase causes myocardial ischemia.

The finding that norepinephrine causes cord necrosis when injected directly into the cord substance is also of dubious significance. Norepinephrine will cause the sloughing of nearly every tissue in the body when injected directly in sufficient quantity. Furthermore, a variety of substances, including histamine, bradykinin, serotonin, will cause hemorrhagic necrosis of the cord after direct installation. Thus, attributing central hemorrhagic necrosis to norepinephrine alone may be unwarranted.

Osterholm's theories spurred the evaluation of a variety of adrenergic-blocking agents in the treatment of experimental spinal injury including alpha-methyltyrosine, phenoxybenzamine, methylsurgide, haloperidol, alpha-methyldopa, Reserpine, 6-hydroxydopamine, disulfiram, fusuric acid, and levodopa. A complete review of the literature that deals with the use of antinorepinephrine, antidopamine, and antiserotonin agents in spinal cord injury is beyond the scope of this chapter but can be found in Osterholm's review. It is sufficient to state that every compound listed here has been found to enhance the motor recovery and histological appearance of the spinal cords of experimental animals following incomplete impact SCI. There have been no reports documenting the use of adrenergic blockades in the treatment of human SCI. From a practical standpoint, despite the impressive experimental literature, the catecholamine theory of SCI has had little impact on the clinical problems of spinal injury.

Naloxone

Faden et al. found that SCI in cats causes the release of beta endorphinlike substances into the bloodstream and reasoned that these substances, which cause significant peripheral vasodilatation, are responsible for the systemic hypotension and the reduced perfusion to the spinal cord that follow SCI.[12,13] Since the endorphins are endogenous opiate compounds, Faden evaluated the effects of administering naloxone, a synthetic opiate antagonist, to cats following an Allen impact injury. He observed that naloxone blocked the hypotension associated with spinal trauma and improved the average modified Tarlov score of the animals treated.[12,13,14] Since that time, other researchers have documented the beneficial effects of the administration of naloxone in improving neurologic outcome in SCI. Furthermore, naloxone has been reported to improve neurologic function in cats subjected to cervical cord injury, even when given four hours after injury.

The exact mechanism of the naloxone effect in SCI is not known. It has been postulated that endogenous opiates play a role in the posttraumatic ischemia that develops following such injuries, and that naloxone, by blocking the influence of these opiates, ameliorates the associated ischemia. Another theory is that naloxone acts by increasing cardiac output to the spinal cord without a significant associated rise in mean systemic pressure. It was noted in the work of Holaday et al., which showed improved cardiac performance in endotoxic and hypovolemic shock, that naloxone administration produced no significant associated increase in mean systemic pressure.[14]

Some investigators have criticized the naloxone studies, however, claiming that researchers in this area have merely demonstrated that cardiac output improves following SCI, improvement that can be achieved in human patients with the administration of fluids or pressors. Thus, naloxone itself may not have any direct action on the injured cord. Moreover, as Faden observes, the administration of naloxone may not be ethical in humans since the drug reverses the pain killing properties of exogenous opiates, such as morphine, which may be necessary to control severe pain in spinal fractures and other associated trauma. Despite these concerns, a multicenter trial of naloxone in the treatment of clinical spinal cord injury is currently underway under the auspices of the National Acute Spinal Cord Injury Study sponsored by the National Institutes of Health.

Thyrotropin-Releasing Hormone

Faden et al., concerned about the potentially pain enhancing properties of naloxone, investigated the effect of thyrotropin-releasing hormone (TRH) on the outcome of experimental SCI in cats. The TRH is known to act as a physiological, antiopiate substance but seems to spare the analgesia system and so Faden's group reasoned that they could obtain the benefits of naloxone using TRH but avoid the antianalgesia associated with its use. In the same experimental system used to evaluate naloxone (600 g cm impact injury in cats followed serially using the modified Tarlov scale), TRH was found to be as effective as naloxone in preventing the hypotension that normally follows SCI and also as effective in improving the modified Tarlov scales of the animals after injury.[14]

The TRH can be criticized in the same manner as was naloxone. It may act only as a pressor agent with no direct effect on the spinal cord. As such, this expensive compound may be of no more benefit than the rapid fluid resuscitation of the SCI patient. Unlike naloxone, however, there is some evidence that thyroid hormones (which are released as a result of TRH administration) have some direct beneficial effect on the injured spinal cord. For example, Tator and Van der Jagt observed an improved recovery in rats following the administration of both T3 and T4.[34]

Unlike naloxone, there have been no human trials of TRH in spinal cord injury. Genetic technology should make large quantities of TRH available in the future, and a trial of this substance in clinical SCI is presently in the planning stages.

Hyperbaric Oxygen

Hyperbaric oxygen, like steroids, is one of the few medical therapies of SCI that has been evaluated in both animal and human trials. In animals, 100 percent oxygen at two to three atm of pressure has been found to be beneficial in enhancing the motor recovery of baboons, sheep, and dogs. The rationale behind the use of hyperbaric oxygen is simple. By increasing the blood oxygen tension, the hypoxic effects that injury induces in the spinal cord (which are secondary to poor blood flow) can be partially reversed.[23,26,35]

Most of the clinical data concerning the use of hyperbaric oxygen in human patients with SCI comes from areas, such as Australia, where deep-sea diving and hyperbaric chambers are prevalent. Unfortunately, all the clinical results reported to date in this field are anecdotal. For example, the study of Jones et al. is typical. These investigators treated seven patients with severe SCI within 12 hours of injury using 2.5 atm of pure oxygen. Of the seven, two died, three remained completely paralyzed, and two had modest motor recovery. However, the two who showed recovery were patients who had incomplete cord injuries from the beginning, so it is not possible to attribute any improvement in their motor function to the hyperbaric oxygen therapy.[23] Without a large number of patients and adequate controls, it is impossible to evaluate the treatment of incompletely injured patients because these patients have unpredictable recovery without any treatment. Thus, the benefits of hyperbaric oxygen treatment in SCI remain open to question.[2]

Proteolytic Enzyme Therapy

Matinian and Andresian reported in the Soviet literature that proteolytic enzymes, such as trypsin or elastase, will allow an almost miraculous recovery of motor function when administered subcutaneously or intramuscularly in rats who have been injured with sharp surgical transection of the spinal cord.[27] This report caused considerable excitement, but investigators in the United States, such as Feringa, have failed to duplicate these findings despite meticulous attempts to reproduce the original techniques employed.[15]

The theory behind the use of proteolytic enzymes in SCI is simple. The Soviet scientists postulated that the only impediment to the regeneration of the transected cord is fibrous scar that forms over the cut ends of the cord. By inhibiting this scar, the regenerating axons can be allowed to seek their end points and restore the continuity of the descending and ascending pathways in the spinal cord.

It is the current consensus of opinion that the Russians used a grossly inadequate technique of spinal cord section that left much of the anterior motor pathways intact. As such, this unusual report must stand as an irreproducible relic in the history of SCI research and the proteolytic enzyme therapy of SCI is currently an inactive topic.

Lidocaine

Kobrine et al. showed that intravenous lidocaine initiated 15 minutes after a balloon compression injury to the spinal cord of cats reduces the pathologic changes seen in the cords at autopsy and permits the recovery of evoked potential transmission in the animals. Their study did not report functional motor recovery in the treated animals. The authors postulate that lidocaine acts by stabilizing neural membranes, preserving axonal conduction, and preventing the leakage of potassium out of injured neurons. Lidocaine has not been used clinically to any extent for human spinal cord injury.[25]

Immunosuppression

Feringa et al. proposed that autoimmunity may hinder regeneration of the wounded spinal cord and has suggested that immunosuppressive drugs may permit an improved outcome following SCI. The central nervous system is generally an immunoprivileged site and neural trauma is often followed by the appearance of antibodies and T-lymphocytes directed against neural proteins and myelin products. Like Matinian and Andresian, Feringa's group felt that recovery is impeded by the inflammatory response of the immune and reticuloendothelial systems to SCI, and they also employed a model using total surgical transection of rat spinal cords. They found that a variety of immunosuppressive agents, including azathioprine and antilymphocyte serum, allow the recovery of evoked potential transmission in some animals.[16]

Unfortunately, these researchers do not provide the same dramatic results supplied by the Russian investigators. The therapy suggested by Feringa's group is so toxic that only the most stunning of results could convince a clinician to try it on human patients. The restoration of electrical potential conduction is not sufficient for the establishment of human trials of immunosuppression in SCI until further animal trials are forthcoming.

Dimethylsulfoxide

Geldered reviews the rationale for the use of dimethylsulfoxide (DMSO) in SCI. He points out that DMSO, like so many other compounds, improves the motor recovery of animals if administered topically after the production of an experimental impact SCI. Dimethylsulfoxide is a diuretic so its use in SCI may mimic the use of urea and mannitol in head injury, i.e., it may act as an antiedema agent. Some authors claim that DMSO enhances oxygen delivery to ischemic tissues, while others claim it has an anti-inflammatory property. No human trials of DMSO in SCI have been reported.[17,24]

Current Medical Therapy

The best current initial medical and pharmacologic therapy of spinal cord injury in children is based on the potentially reversible pathophysiological changes that occur related to reduction in spinal cord blood flow.

Blood pressure should be vigorously supported and mild hypertension induced to ensure adequate spinal cord blood flow for at least the first 12 to 24 hours following injury. Fluid resuscitation is a keystone to the initial therapy. Even in the absence of associated injury, however, it may be very difficult to maintain an adequate perfusion pressure in the presence of vasogenic spinal shock. Fluid resuscitation should consist of an appropriate combination of crystalloid and colloid solutions, depending on the presence of associated injury. In many instances, lactated Ringer's solution is the best initial fluid to employ. If, despite adequate fluid replacement, as evidenced by central venous pressure readings in the range of 10 to 12 cm of water, the blood pressure cannot be normalized or elevated slightly, pressors such as dopamine should be instituted.

As spinal cord blood flow is dependent not only on perfusion pressure but blood rheology as well, it is important to consider measures to reduce blood viscosity, thereby increasing perfusion. Decreased viscosity can be achieved maximally with blood hematocrits in the range of 33 percent to 37 percent. Use of plasmanate, Albumisol, or other similar colloid agents can be helpful in this regard.

Maintenance of adequate tissue oxygenation is also important in the first hours following spinal cord injury. Inadequate oxygenation of the injured regions of the cord will only hasten the pathophysiological cascade that occurs. Careful attention must be paid to airway maintenance, intubation, assisted mechanical ventilation if necessary, and maintenance of satisfactory blood pO_2 levels.

Steroids are still used routinely in the majority of spinal cord injury centers for the treatment of acute spinal cord injury. The clinical trials remain inconclusive, but the basis for using steroids is quite substantial, and the limited amount of morbidity from the short-term use of these agents warrants their continued use in spinal cord injury until definitive studies prove that they have no benefit whatsoever.

CONCLUSIONS

Several conclusions are possible from the currently available literature and research on the pharmacotherapy of human and animal spinal cord injury.

Only steroids and hyperbaric oxygen have been used to any great extent in human patients. Trials of hyperbaric oxygen therapy are anecdotal and uninterpretable, while the one randomized trial of steroids in human spinal cord injury found no benefit of high dose therapy over low dose therapy. No trial of steroids versus placebo in spinal cord injury has been published, but one cooperative study sponsored by the National Acute Spinal Cord Injury Study is underway at the present time.

Animal models of spinal cord injury generally use impact injuries that are carefully titrated to give the appearance of a severe injury but without the sequela of complete cord injury. Thus, nearly all of the impact animal studies that have been published evaluate only the pharmacotherapy of incomplete injuries. Those studies that investigated complete injuries report improvement only in terms of improved evoked potential conduction or an improved histological appearance of the cord following injury.

The only study reporting motor recovery following a complete cord lesion is the Russian trial of proteolytic enzyme therapy in rats, which has never been reproduced and, thus, is probably invalid.

The fact that such an incredible variety of agents has produced clinical benefit in animal impact injury models, while no medical therapy of human spinal cord injury is at hand raises the suspicion that current animal models of spinal cord injury are not adequate simulations of human fracture dislocation spinal injuries.

There is some hope on the horizon, however. Naloxone, TRH, and lidocaine are substances that are relatively nontoxic, have shown to effect great neurologic improvement following spinal cord injury in animal models, and have yet to be evaluated in a clinical setting. The clinical trial for naloxone is currently underway under the auspices of the National Spinal Cord Injury Study. Perhaps further clinical trials will offer more answers to the difficult clinical problems posed by spinal cord injury.

REFERENCES

1. Allen AR: Surgery of experimental lesions of spinal cord equivalent to crush injury of fracture dislocation of spinal column. Preliminary report. *JAMA* 57:878–880, 1911.
2. Black P, Markowitz RS: Experimental spinal cord injury in monkeys: Comparison of steroids and local hypothermia. *Surg Forum* 22:409–411, 1971.
3. Bracken MB, Cullins WF, Freeman DF, et al: Efficacy of methylprednisolone in acute spinal cord injury. *JAMA* 251:45–52, 1984.
4. Campbell JB, Decrescito V, Tomasula JJ et al: Effects of antifibrinolytic and steroid therapy on the contused spinal cord of cats. *J Neurosurg* 40:726–733, 1974.
5. Campbell JB, Decrescito V, Tomasula JJ, et al: Experimental treatment of spinal cord contusion in the cat. *Surg Neurol* 1:102–106, 1973.
6. Conn HO, Blitzer BL: Non-association of adrenocorticoid steroid therapy and peptic ulcer. *N Engl J Med* 294:473–480, 1976.
7. Delatorre JC, Johnson CM, Gould DJ, et al: Pharmacologic treatment and evaluation of permanent experimental spinal cord trauma. *Neurology* 25:508–514, 1975.

8. Delatorre JC: Spinal cord injury, Review of basic and applied research. *Spine* 6:315–334, 1981.
9. Ducker TB: Experimental injury of the spinal cord, in Vinkin PJ, Bruyn, GW (eds) *Handbook of Clinical Neurology*. Amsterdam, North Holland, 1976, vol 25, pp 9–26.
10. Ducker TB, Hamit HF: Experimental treatments of acute spinal cord injury. *J Neurosurg* 30:693–697, 1969.
11. Eidelberg E, Staton E, Watkins CJ, et al: Treatment of experimenntal spinal cord injury in ferrets. *Surg Neurol* 6:243–246, 1976.
12. Faden AI, Jacobs TP, Mougey E, et al: Endorphins and experimental spinal injury: Therapeutic effect of naloxone. *Ann Neurol* 10:326–332, 1981.
13. Faden AI, Jacobs TP, Holaday JW: Opiate antagonist improves neurologic recovery after spinal injury. *Science* 211:493–494, 1981.
14. Faden AI, Jacobs TP, Holaday JW: Thyrotropin-releasing hormone improves neurologic recovery after spinal trauma in cats. *N Engl J Med* 305:1063–1067, 1981.
15. Feringa ER, Kowalski TF, Vahlsing HL, et al: Enzyme treatment of spinal cord transected rats. *Ann Neurol* 5:203–206, 1979.
16. Feringa ER, Kowalski TF, Vahlsing HL, et al: Immunosuppressive treatment to enhance spinal cord regeneration in rats. *Neurology* 24:287–293, 1974.
17. Geldered JB: Hyperbaric oxygen and dimethylsulfoxide therapy following spinal cord injury, in Kao CC et al (eds) *Spinal Cord Reconstruction*. New York, Raven Press, 1983, pp 245–259.
18. Green BA, Kahn T, Klose KJ: A comparative study of steroid therapy in acute experimental spinal cord injury. *Surg Neurol* 13:91–97, 1980.
19. Hall ED, Braughler JM: Acute effects of intravenous glucocorticoid treatment on the in vitro peroxidation of cats' spinal cord tissue. *Exp Neurol* 73:321–324, 1981.
20. Hall ED, Braughler JM: Glucocorticoid mechanisms in acute spinal cord injury: A review and therapeutic rationale. *Surg Neurol* 18:320–327, 1982.
21. Hansebout RR: A comprehensive review of methods of improving cord recovery after acute spinal cord injury, in Tator CH (ed) *Early Management of Acute Spinal Cord Injury*. New York, Raven Press, 1982, pp 181–196.
22. Hendemen LS, Shellenbarger MK, Gordon JH: Studies on experimental spinal cord trauma, Part 1: Alterations of catecholamine levels. *J Neurosurg* 40:37–43, 1974.
23. Jones RF, Unsworth IP, Marosszkey JE: Hyperbaric oxygen in acute spinal injuries in humans. *Med J Aust* 2:573–575, 1978.
24. Kajihara K, Kawanga H, Delatorre JC, et al: Dimethylsulfoxide in the treatment of acute spinal cord injury. *Surg Neurol* 1:16–23, 1973.
25. Kobrine AI, Evans DE, Legrys DC, et al: Effect of lidocaine on experimental spinal cord injury. *J Neurosurg* 60:595–601, 1984.
26. Kuchner EF, Hansebout RR: Combined steroid and hypothermia

treatment of experimental spinal cord injuries. *Surg Neurol* 6:371–376, 1976.

27. Matinian LA, Andresian AS: Enzyme therapy in organic lesions of the spinal cord. *Translation of the Brain Information Services*, 1976, pp 42–68.
28. Means ED, Douglas DK, Walters, TR, Kalif L: Effect of methylprednisolone in compression trauma to the feline spinal cord. *J Neurosurg* 55:200–208, 1981.
29. Mendenhall HV, Litwak P, Yturraspe DJ, et al: Aggressive pharmacologic and surgical treatment in dogs and cats. *J Am Vet Med Assoc* 168:1026–1031, 1976.
30. Osterholm JL, Matthews GJ: Altered norepinephrine metabolism following experimental spinal cord injury. Part I Relationship to hemorrhagic necrosis in postwounding neurological deficits. *J Neurosurg* 36:386–394, 1972.
31. Osterholm JL: The pathophysiological response to spinal cord injury: The current status of related research. *J Neurosurg* 40:5–33, 1974.
32. Parker AJ, Smith CW: Functional recovery from spinal cord trauma following dexamethasone and chlorpromazine therapy in dogs. *Res Vet Sci* 21:246–247, 1976.
33. Tarlov IM: Spinal Cord Compression: Mechanism of Paralysis and Treatment. Springfield, IL, CC Thomas, 1957, p 147.
34. Tator CH, Van der Jagt, EHC: Effect of exogenous thyroid hormones on functional recovery of the rat after acute spinal cord compression injury. *J Neurosurg* 53:381–394, 1980.
35. Yeo, JB, Stabback AS, MCKenzie B: A study of the effects of hyperbaric oxygen on the experimental spinal cord injury. *Med J Aust* 2:145–147, 1977.

Chapter 7

SURGICAL MANAGEMENT OF SPINAL CORD INJURIES

James E. Wilberger, Jr., Parviz Baghai, and Mahnaz Tadjziechy

The role of surgery in the treatment of spinal fractures and spinal cord injuries is controversial. Considerable disagreement exists regarding the place of surgery in such injuries and, should surgical treatment be decided on, what should be done and when.[8,9,17,18,23,27,29] The major goal in the surgical treatment of these injuries is the restoration and maintenance of normal anatomical relationships between the spinal cord and spinal canal and the return of the patient to the fullest possible activity in the shortest period of time. All clinicians are in agreement as to the absolute necessity for immediate immobilization and stabilization of fractures and dislocations of the spine and subsequent surgical intervention for the fusion of unstable fractures and dislocations.[7,17,20,23] However, the indications for acute surgical intervention in spinal cord injury are less clear. Patients recommended for acute surgery have included those with preservation of some distal neurologic function who fail to improve or demonstrate evidence of progressive neurologic deficit. The presence of an incomplete myelopathy with persistent spinal cord deformity and complete myelopathy when the possibility exists for recovery of some additional nerve root function also have been used as indications for surgical intervention.[23,31] Once a course of surgery has been chosen, special consideration must be given to the operative approaches to the spine and the anesthetic management of these patients, which may be quite different than those commonly used in adults with similar injuries.

SPINAL STABILITY

The evaluation for instability is the most important determining factor in the decision-making process regarding the operative or nonoperative management of spinal fractures. Stability is defined as the absence of any abnormal mobility between any pair of vertebrae when lateral x-ray films are taken in flexion and extension at the conclusion of the treatment of a fracture or fracture dislocation. Stability, when applied to an acute fracture or dislocation, refers to the predicted ultimate stability of the spine following appropriate therapy and not the immediate state. Predicted stability as a basis for therapy in specific injuries has often been the basis for arguments between advocates of surgery and those for long-term orthotic management of spinal fractures.[7,25,30]

The anatomical structures that are important in providing stability have been evaluated by various investigators. It appears that the disc as well as the other soft tissue structures and the posterior element complex of the spine are quite important in providing stability. White et al. concluded that all posterior structures and one anterior structure, or all anterior structures and one posterior structure must be damaged to create laboratory instability, and if all the anterior or all the posterior structures have been destroyed, clinical instability will result.[32] One may attempt to evaluate the degree of instability by analyzing the pattern of fracture as well as the forces involved in producing the injury. Holdsworth described specific fracture patterns and grouped injuries into those which were stable or unstable.[16] The wedge-compression fracture, burst injury, and most extension injuries were considered to be stable. Unstable fractures include all dislocations and subluxations. White et al. have compiled a list of specific factors that may play a role in assessing stability. They have included injuries to the anterior and posterior column, as well as factors that relate to displacement, such as sagittal translation of greater than 3.5 mm, flexion of greater than 11 degrees, and distraction of greater than 1.7 mm.

The forces involved in creating spinal column injuries also play a role in determining the degree of instability. Flexion and vertical compression, flexion and rotation, and vertical compression and extension are the most important forces producing disruption of the spinal column. A vertical compression fracture will lead to a bursting injury of the body, leaving the posterior elements relatively intact. If significant flexion and rotation have occurred, not only will the vertebral body be crushed, but rupture of the posterior ligamentous complex can also occur. Dislocations are also unstable due to damage of the disc and complete disruptions of the soft tissues posteriorly. Radiographically, the special points which should always be looked for are the presence or absence of separation of the spinous processes, which implies significant posterior ligamentous disruption, and the presence of dislocation or fracture of the articular processes.[3]

Thus, while varying definitions of stability have been used, most authors agree that stability is dependent on the degree of damage to the posterior ligamentous complex. Cheshire defines stability as the absence of abnormal mobility on flexion-extension stress films. In a study of 212 patients with cervical injuries, he found an overall instability rate of 4.8 percent to 7.3 percent for various fractures, but found a very high 21 percent instability rate when the posterior ligamentous complex was involved.[7] White et al. define stability as the ability of the spine to maintain vertebral relationships under physiological loads, so that neither neurologic damage nor deformity with excess pain occurs.[32] The objective of surgical and nonsurgical management of these injuries is to maintain normal vertebral relationships.

ACUTE SURGERY FOR SPINAL CORD INJURY

The primary goals of the early management of children with spinal cord injury are the preservation of injured but still potentially viable neural tissue and the prevention of further spinal cord injury. Both objectives can be achieved initially by the use of spinal traction for immobilization and reduction of fractures. However, the question of whether early surgical intervention for decompression of the spinal cord with secondary stabilization leads to a significant improvement in neurologic prognosis has been debated for decades. Considerable disagreement exists over the place of acute surgery in 1) children with incomplete cord injury who have radiographically significant ongoing spinal cord deformity in spite of fracture reduction; 2) those children with complete spinal cord injury and reducible or unreducible bony injuries.[28]

Bedbrook, in 1976, asserted that surgery is rarely indicated in spinal cord injury.[2] However, in 1979, Tator and Rowed advocated surgery for an incomplete injury with persistent myelographic compression, and for progression of neurologic deficits. These authors saw no proven indications for surgery in those patients with immediate complete neurologic deficits.[30] Ranshoff et al., in 1979, developed acute surgical indications based on myelography. If amipaque myelography showed near or total block due to either external compression or to intramedullary spinal cord swelling, he felt surgery was indicated. He described 30 patients with incomplete lesions, 17 had surgery on the first few days following injury. Eight of these ambulated without braces or crutches after rehabilitation.[24] Carol et al. developed acute surgical indications based on the performance of minimyelography on all cord injured patients. While in traction, immediately following admission, 3 to 6 cc's of Pantopaque were injected via C1-2 puncture. Complete myelographic block or a significant anterior or posterior impression consistent with the bony or neurologic level or both were taken as indications for immediate surgery.[5] Recently, amipaque myelography in conjunction with computerized tomographic scanning has been used extensively in the presence of neurologic deficits. This technique gives excellent visualization of bony, disc, and spinal cord abnormalities.[10] The advent of magnetic resonance imaging, with its ability to precisely define anatomic abnormalities may, in the future, obviate all other types of studies in the acute evaluation of spinal cord injury.

Assuming appropriate indications for acute surgical intervention can be established, what are the results of such surgery? In 1956, Comarr reviewed 858 patients with spinal cord injury from 1947 to 1956. Acute laminectomies for spinal cord decompression were performed on 579 of these patients. Postoperative improvement was noted in 16 percent of the laminectomy patients, with 8 percent becoming ambulatory. Of the 279 patients not subjected to acute surgery, 29 percent improved and 16 percent became ambulatory.[8,9] Morgan et al., in 1971, reviewed 230 patients from 1954 to 1968. Seventy of the patients had incomplete cord lesions and, of these, 42 underwent immediate laminectomy. Twenty-two (52 percent) of these patients lost function following surgery, and ten developed complete lesions. Fourteen patients improved following the surgery.[21] Heiden et al. reviewed 356 patients treated from 1963 to 1972. Complete spinal cord injury was present in 193, of whom 121 underwent surgery. No improvement was seen in any patient who had surgery, regardless of timing. Similarly, there was no significant difference between patients who had posterior laminectomies performed and those who underwent anterior decompressive procedures. Of the remaining 78 patients who did not undergo surgery, two regained useful motor function in the legs. Heiden singled out 12 patients with anterior cord syndrome, five were treated with surgery but did not improve. Three of the seven patients not operated on showed significant neurologic improvement.[15] Finally, Carol et al. reported their surgical results in 1980. Fifty-eight patients underwent minimyelography and met strict surgical criteria for early intervention. Five were operated on acutely. Three of the 5 had extruded discs. Of these, two improved neurologically at a faster rate than predicted postoperatively. One patient had no structural abnormality at surgery, and one patient developed an ascending neurologic level and died. Thus, of the five patients operated on acutely, two improved faster than predicted.[5] Results such as these have led some to state emphatically that acute decompressive surgery has no place in the management of spinal cord injury even in the presence of incomplete lesions. However, many of the older studies relied solely on posterior laminectomy as the form of decompression when in the vast majority of instances of spinal cord injury, the primary pathology responsible for ongoing compression is anterior. However, as noted in both the Heiden and Carol studies, anterior approaches were frequently used without producing a significant difference in outcome. Thus, the advocates of immediate surgery for spinal cord injury are finding little support for their position. However, clinical studies are still underway in many of the leading spinal cord injury centers to seek to definitively answer this question.

Stable or unstable thoracolumbar fractures require a somewhat different approach on an immediate basis. Injuries at this level may include elements of the spinal cord (conus medullaris) or peripheral nerves (cauda equina) either singly or in combination. It has been fairly definitively shown that incomplete injuries in this region may show significant neurologic improvement after relief of bony compression of the neural elements.[11,16,30]

SURGERY FOR SPINE STABILIZATION

Scant information exists as to the indications, techniques, and results for spine stabilization following fractures and dislocations in children. From 1958 to 1968, Toronto's Sick Children's Hospital reviewed 13 cases of cervical fusion in children 2 to 15 years of age. On the basis of their results, they advocated a one-level posterior cervical fusion at the site of injury to preserve maximum physiological mobility and to allow for growth. All but three of the cases reported were said to have a stable cervical spine following one operation. Two children required one additional operation before the spine was stable, and the spine in the third child still was not fused after a second operation.[23] Boston Children's Hospital reported on six children who underwent fusion for instability secondary to trauma. Ages ranged from five months to nine years. Four of the six had hypermobility without evidence of a fracture. Autogenous grafting was used posteriorly in all, with wire fixation used in four of the six. Their results also suggested that limited posterior fusion was effective in providing stabilization.[22] The Mayo Clinic reported 23 surgical procedures on 158 spinal cord injured children for stabilization, but the results of their procedures were not described.[1] Children's Hospital in Seattle reported on 42 cases of spine instability secondary to trauma, nine of whom required fusion. The fusions were described as being successful in every case, but the details were not given.[18]

Both anterior and posterior approaches to the cervical spine have been recommended for decompression and reduction of fractures and dislocations with subsequent stabilization. Advocates of the anterior approach feel that it restores the biomechanics of the spine and reduces the inci-

dence of kyphosis, while at the same time allowing for removal of any bony or disc elements that may be a source for
ongoing spinal cord compression. The anterior approach
has been recommended primarily for burst or teardrop fractures. Stauffer and Kelly reported a series of 16 children and
adolescents treated by anterior interbody fusion for various
types of cervical fracture dislocations. All 16 were found to
be unstable postoperatively, with the development of angular deformities presumably secondary to incompetence of
the posterior ligamentous structures. Of these patients,
three suffered progressive neurologic deterioration. This
led Stauffer and Kelly to adamantly state that anterior fusion should never be performed as a primary surgical treatment for stabilization of cervical fractures in children.[29]
Many other authors are of the same opinion. It has been
shown that surgical elevation of the anterior longitudinal
ligament and exposure of the incompletely developed central vertebral cartilage and ossification centers may cause
widespread fusion to occur anteriorly.

Thus, it would appear that when fusion is necessary,
the posterior approach with autogenous bone grafting with
or without wire fixation is the safest route to stabilization of
cervical fractures in children. The more limited the fusion,
the greater the maintenance of physiological mobility and
tolerance for growth. When the posterior approach is
utilized, multiple level laminectomies should be avoided as
this in itself can result in increased instability, even if fusion is performed. When fusing posteriorly in a young
child, it is often necessary only to expose the posterior vertebral elements subperiosteally before laying in the bone
graft. Fusion is rapidly accomplished in this fashion and
wiring may be unnecessary. However, a similar caution
applies in posterior fusions as it does in anterior fusions;
that is, the exposure of more vertebrae than necessary may
lead to multiple level creeping fusion.

Cervical fractures that should be considered unstable in

children requiring operative stabilization include the following:

1. Atlanto-occipital dislocation—Because of ligamentous disruption, fusion from the occiput to C1 and C2 is required.
2. Atlantoaxial rotary fixation—Significant ligamentous disruption requires a C1, C2 fusion for this problem.
3. Compression burst fractures
4. Fractures with dislocations of the lower cervical spine

Fractures that are generally stable and rarely require surgical intervention include the following:

1. Atlas fractures
2. Dens fractures
3. Hangman's fractures

Unstable fractures of the thoracolumbar spine include the following:

1. Burst fractures
2. Hyperextension with compression
3. Hyperflexion with rotation fractures

When untreated, these thoracolumbar fractures will show continuing displacement, angular deformity, and development of scoliosis. Severe chronic pain and progressive neurologic deficits may also occur. Open reduction, internal fixation, and fusion are required. Harrington distraction or compression rods have proved to be an excellent means of internal fixation for these types of fractures. Severely comminuted anterior fractures may require an anterior or anteriolateral approach to the spine for removal of compres-

sive bone fragments and subsequent fusion. If posterior dislocation is present without significant bony disruption,
Harrington distraction rods often may be used effectively to
achieve reduction.

If surgery for stabilization of spinal fractures is indicated, it is generally recommended to wait at least seven to
ten days after an injury as early surgery is associated with a
high pulmonary morbidity. This is especially true in high
cervical injuries where pulmonary reserve may be minimal.

POSTERIOR APPROACHES AND FUSIONS

The posterior approach to the cervical spine is the generally preferred method of stabilization for fracture-
dislocations in children. Similarly, this approach is generally best for unstable thoracolumbar injuries. Immediate
stability can be accomplished by using wire (cervical spine)
or rods (thoracolumbar spine), and long-term stability can
be ensured utilizing autogenous bone grafting. Various
types of wiring (sublaminal, interspinous, interfacetal) and
rods (Harrington compression and distraction, Luque) have
been developed. Bony fusion can be accomplished using
iliac crest, fibula, or rib. The technique of wiring or fusion
selected depends on the anatomy and biomechanics of the
bony injury involved.[11,20,25,27,33]

Occipitocervical Fusion

As the majority of neck motion in flexion, extension,
and rotation occurs at the occipito-atlanto-axial level, an
occipitocervical fusion should be reserved for those situations in which extreme instability exists at this level. One of
the few indications for this type of fusion in children is
atlanto-occipital dislocation in which a complete disruption of supporting ligamentous elements has occurred. As

noted previously (Chapter 4) such an injury should be immediately stabilized in a halo cast. The surgery is performed
with the child in the halo cast in the prone position. The
skin in the posterior cervical region can be infiltrated with a
small amount of a 1% solution of Xylocaine with 1:200,000
epinephrine so as to minimize skin bleeding. A skin incision is made in the midline, extending from the external
occipital protoberance to C4 or C5. The fascia and muscles
are dissected subperiosteally to expose the suboccipital region, the foramen magnum, and the altas as well as the
spinous processes and laminae of C2 and C3. Careful sharp
dissection must be carried out around the foramen magnum
and the posterior arch of C1 so as to avoid the vertebral
artery and venous plexus, which pass over the lateral portions of C1 to enter the foramen magnum. Wire fusion can
then be accomplished by drilling two holes in the suboccipital bone—one on either side of the midline. A 20-gauge
braided wire is then passed between the holes, under the
laminae of C1 and C2, and twisted securely. Care must be
taken to ensure the easy passage of the wire under C1 and
C2 and the wire must be tightened sufficiently so as to prevent impingement on the spinal canal (Fig. 1). Corticocancellous bone strips are then taken from the iliac crest and
placed laterally from the occiput to C2. Alternately, the
bone strips may be wired in place as well. The child is then
maintained in the halo cast until complete bone fusion has
occurred—generally 8 to 12 weeks (Fig. 2).

Atlantoaxial Fusion

Atlantoaxial fusion in children may be indicated in
several instances. Severe atlantoaxial rotary fixation in
which significant ligamentous disruption has occurred is
an unstable injury requiring fusion of C1 and C2. While
dens fractures generally heal quite well with immobilization, occasionally nonunion will occur requiring C1-2 fu-

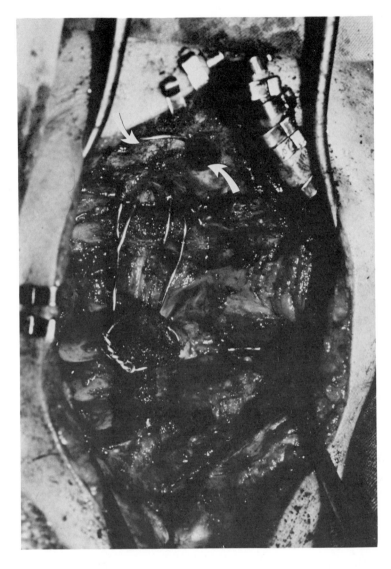

Figure 1. Photograph demonstrating passage of a 20-gauge wire between two holes in the occiput (arrows) and under the laminae of C1 and C2 to provide for occipitocervical fusion.

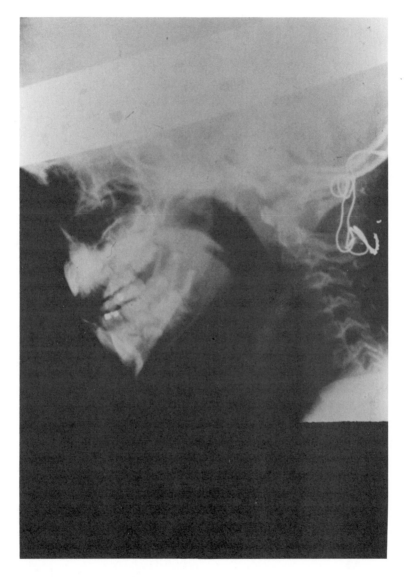

Figure 2. Lateral radiograph one month following surgery showing positioning of the wire and beginning ossification of the bony fusion between the occiput and C3.

sion. Also congenital anomalies at the C1-2 level, such as os odontoideum, may require such a fusion.

The approach to the upper cervical spine for C1-2 fusion is the same as that for occipitocervical fusion. The head is held in fixation with either Gardner-Wells tongs or a pin-vise three-point head holder before the child is turned into the prone position. Once the occiput and C1-2 are exposed, one of two approaches to wiring and fusion can be taken—Brooks fusion or Gallie fusion. With Gallie fusion a U-shaped piece of 20-gauge braided wire is passed under the midline of the posterior arch of C1, then swung back, and secured under the spinous process of C2. An H-shaped piece of corticocancellous bone is then held in position by the wire between C1 and C2 (Figs. 3 and 4).[4] With the Brooks fusion, 24-gauge braided wires are placed under the lamine of C2 and the posterior arch of C1—two on each side of the midline—and secured around corticocancellous bone

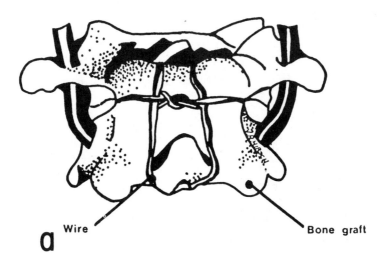

Wire   **Bone graft**

a

Figure 3A. *Gallie fusion involves placing a wire under the arch of C1 and securing it under the spinous processes of C2 (a). An H-shaped piece of iliac crest graft is then secured between C1 and C2 and the wire twisted (b).*

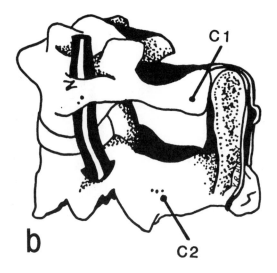

Figure 3B.

grafts placed between C1 and C2 (Fig. 5).[12] Particular care must be taken not to allow passage of the wire or its final position to impinge on the spinal canal. After fusion is accomplished, the child should be kept immobilized in a halo cast or cervicothoracic brace for 8 to 12 weeks.

Lower Cervical Interspinous Fusion

Fusion in the lower cervical region in children is indicated in any situation of a fracture-dislocation resulting in instability (see spinal stability this chapter). Rogers is credited for first describing the technique of interspinous fusion for such injuries.[25] Prior to Rogers' description of the technique, almost all of these injuries were treated by long-term immobilization. The prerequisite for interspinous wiring and fusion is intact posterior elements. It is generally best suited to those situations in which subluxation is primarily due to ligamentous injury.

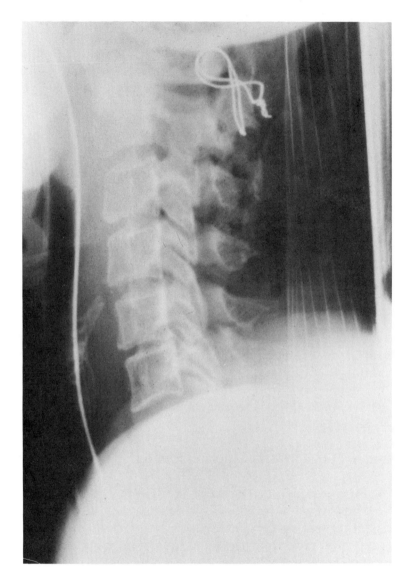

Figure 4. *Lateral radiograph of a Gallie fusion for an odontoid fracture.*

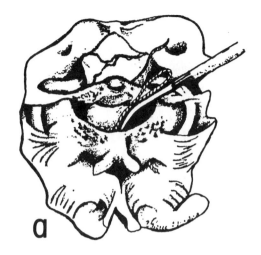

Figure 5A. Brooks fusion involves passage of wire beneath the laminae of C2 and the posterior arch of C1 (a), securing iliac crest grafts between C1 and C2 (b) and tightening the wires to hold the grafts in place (c).

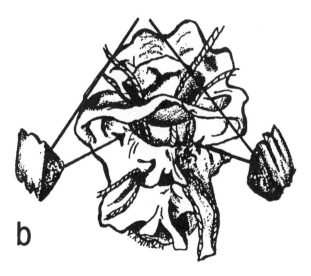

Figure 5B.

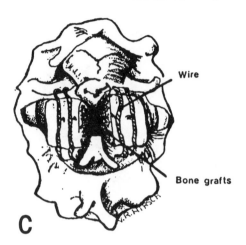

C

Figure 5C.

For interspinous fusion, the child is operated on in the prone position with the head fixed in tongs or pins. Infiltration of the skin with Xylocaine with epinephrine aids in minimizing blood loss. A midline incision is made from C2 to C7 and carried down through the subcutaneous tissue to the fascia. Paracervical musculature and fascia are then dissected subperiosteally to expose spinous processes, laminae, and facets of the involved levels. With significant subluxation, there is often separation of the interspinous and interlaminar ligaments (Fig. 6). Thus, care must be taken during dissection not to enter any dura that may be exposed. A high speed drill is then used to make a through-and-through hole through the base of the spinous process of the subluxed vertebra. The hole can be enlarged with a towel clip. A second hole is drilled at the base of the spinous process of the next lowest vertebra. A 20-gauge wire is then passed from one hole to the next and tightened. If necessary, a third vertebra can be included in the wiring. Strips of corticocancellous iliac crest bone can then be positioned over the lateral aspects of the laminae and facets of

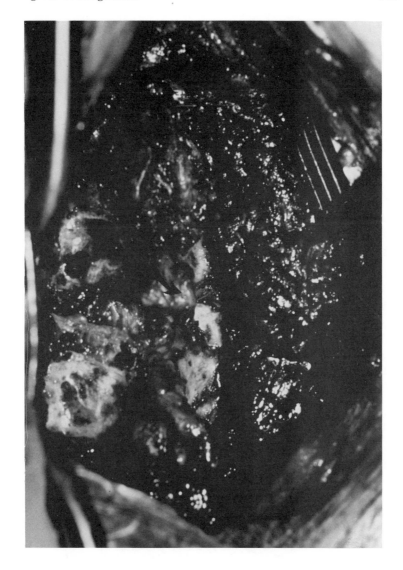

Figure 6. Separation of interspinous and interlaminar ligaments (arrow) in a patient with C3-4 subluxation.

the involved levels (Fig. 7). Extreme caution must be used in drilling the holes and wire passing so as not to injure underlying spinal canal contents. External fixation with a halo cast or cervicothoracic brace must be maintained for 8 to 12 weeks until bony union occurs (Fig. 8).

Cervical Interfacetal Fusion

If the posterior elements are disrupted secondary to injury or are missing due to prior laminectomy, then interspinous wiring is not possible. In such situations interfacetal fusion is indicated.

The approach to the cervical spine for interfacetal fusion is the same as that described for interspinous fusion. However, the facets to be fused must be carefully dissected so as to prevent injury to the laterally placed vertebral artery

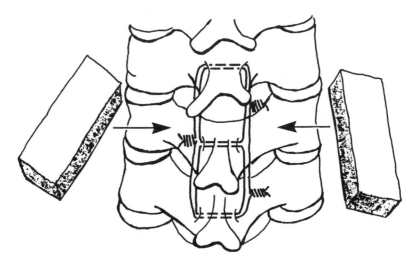

Figure 7. With interspinous wiring the wire is passed between holes drilled at the base of the spinous processes of the involved spinal levels. Iliac crest bone graft can then be laid down over the lateral masses to provide for fusion.

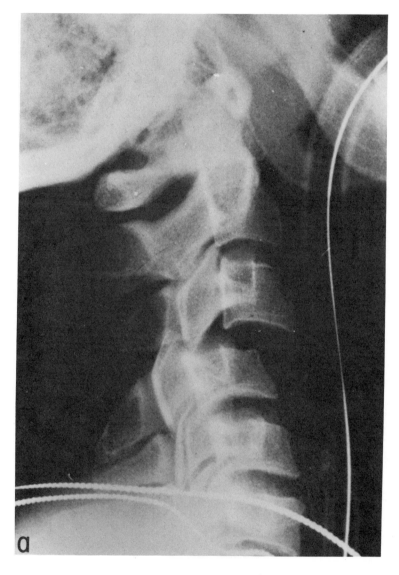

Figure 8A. *Lateral radiographs of a child with C3-4 subluxations (a) which was reduced and fused with interspinous wiring and iliac crest graft (b).*

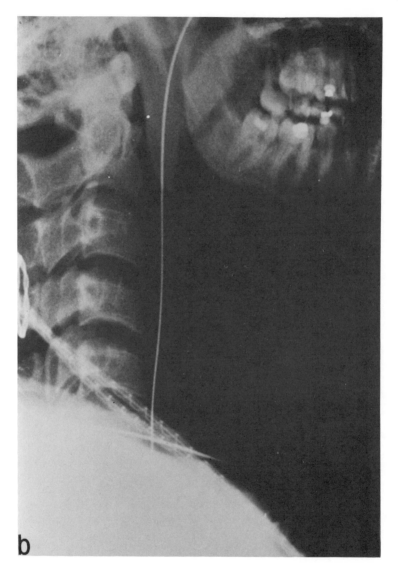

Figure 8B.

and vein. Once the facet joint space is cleared of the joint capsule, a high speed drill is used to place holes through the superior facets bilaterally of the levels to be fused.

Braided 24-gauge stainless steel wire can then be passed from facet to facet and tightened. Strips of corticocancellous iliac crest graft can then be placed between the facets. Alternately, the bone graft may be wired in place over the facets (Fig. 9). Cervical immobilization for 8 to 12 weeks is necessary to ensure bony fusion.

Thoracolumbar Fusion

Like other fractures, thoracolumbar injuries must be assessed in terms of stability. If the fragments of a fracture are

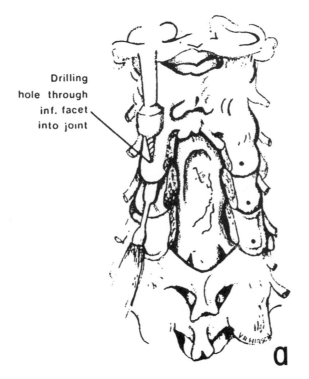

Drilling hole through inf. facet into joint

Figure 9A. *Interfacetal fusion involves wiring between the facets of the involved levels and securing corticocancellous iliac crest grafts over the facets to accomplish fusion (a and b).*

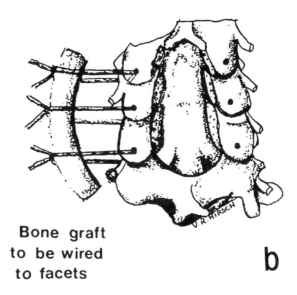

**Bone graft
to be wired
to facets**

b

Figure 9B.

likely to move during healing, the fracture is considered unstable. In general, a greater than 25 percent compression fracture is acutely and chronically unstable and operative fusion is indicated. The development of the Harrington rod has helped alter the surgical perspective on these fractures. The rods act as an internal splint, but more importantly, provide distraction force to restore contour and alignment to the spinal canal and relieve compression (Fig. 10). The combination of neurosurgical decompression and Harrington rod distraction appears to provide the setting for maximum return of neurologic function as well as early ambulation and rehabilitation.[27,30,33]

The currently favored surgical approach for the treatment of thoracolumbar burst-compression fractures in which there is significant spinal canal encroachment by bony fragments is the posterolateral approach. The patient is placed prone on rolls or a frame to allow for hyperextension of the back. The skin incision is made in the midline

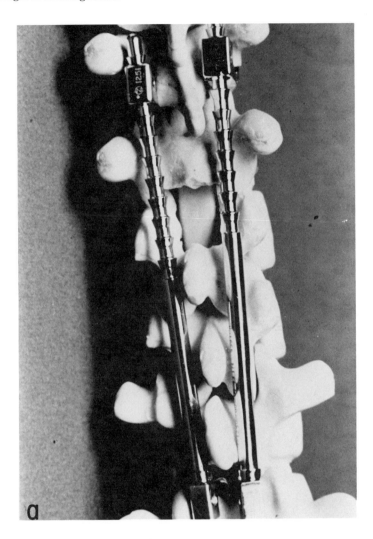

Figure 10A. Ap (a) and lateral (b) views of Harrington rod apparatus in place on a spine model.

and must be long enough to allow visualization of at least two complete laminae and facets above and below the level of the fracture. In many instances, hematoma is encountered

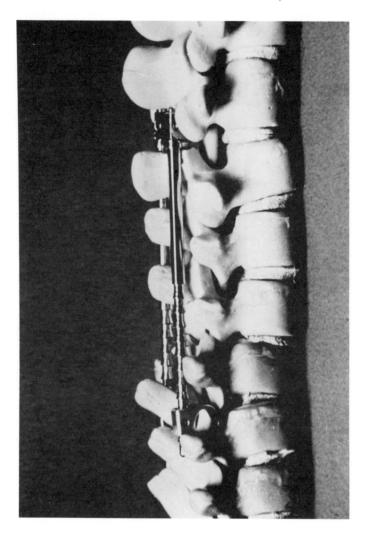

Figure 10B.

in the subcutaneous tissues (Fig. 11). Initially, a sub-
periosteal dissection of the paravertebral muscles is carried
out. The exposure of the fracture site is best performed by
sharp dissection rather than electrocauterization to avoid
injury to any exposed dural or neural elements. The

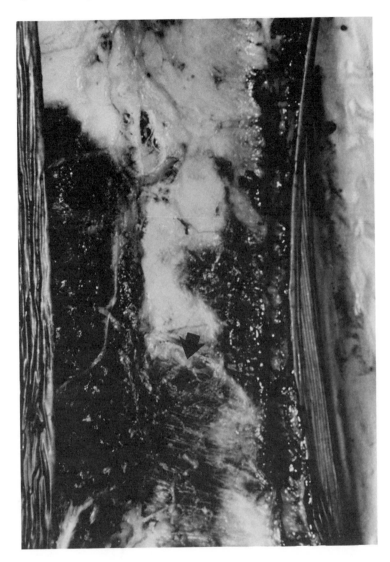

Figure 11. Photograph of a large subcutaneous hematoma (arrows) overlying an L2 compression fracture.

paravertebral muscles are then further mobilized laterally to expose the zygapophysial joints. The fractured vertebral body is then approached by using a high speed drill to remove the lateral aspect of the lamina and the entire pedicle of the involved level. A curette can then be used to enter the vertebral body and remove the posterior bony pieces that are compressing the spinal canal (Fig. 12). Subsequently, Harrington distraction rods are placed. Hooks are placed bilaterally under the laminae two levels above the fracture and bilaterally over the superior aspect of the laminae two levels below the fracture site. The rods are then inserted and secured in position. Corticocancellous iliac crest bone is then laid down laterally. The child should be kept in a molded plastic or plaster body jacket for 10 to 12 weeks until the bony fusion is accomplished (Fig. 13).

An alternate technique of Harrington rod fusion involves the use of sublaminar wires. Eighteen-gauge stainless steel wires are passed under each lamina over which

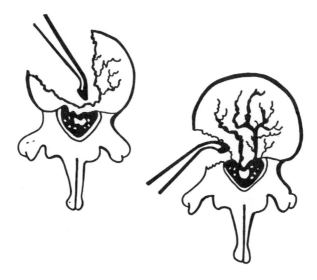

Figure 12. The posteriolateral approach to thoracolumbar burst fractures involves drilling away the lateral aspect of the lamina and pedicle and subsequent direct removal of any compressive bony elements from the spinal canal.

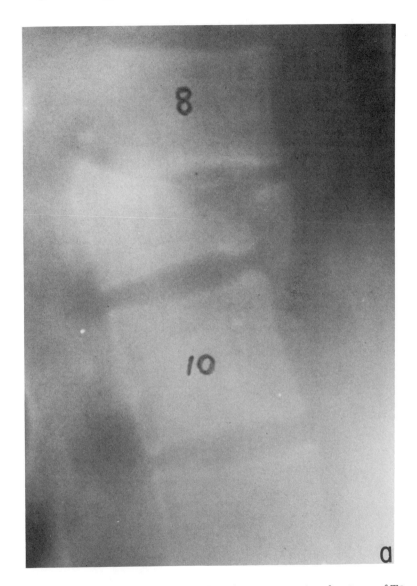

Figure 13A. Lateral radiographs of a compression fracture of T9 with significant posterior displacement (a). Harrington distraction rods have produced normal realignment (b).

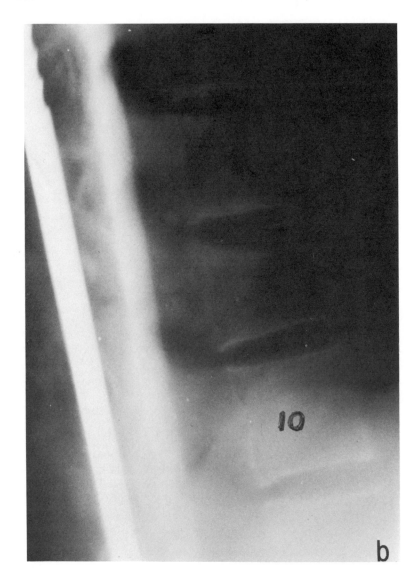

Figure 13B.

the rods pass. The wires are then secured over the rods. It is felt that this technique enhances stability and prevents pulling out or failure of the rods (Fig. 14).

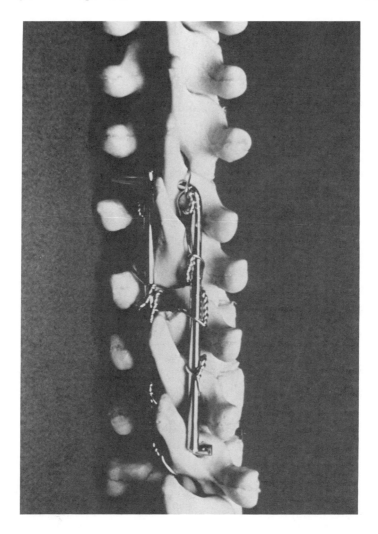

Figure 14. A model spine demonstrating Luque rod fusion with sublaminar wires.

Anterior Approaches and Fusions

The anterior cervical approach to the spine provides an excellent means of exposing the vertebral bodies and intervertebral discs from C3 to T2. Similarly, transthoracic and transabdominal routes can be taken to the anterior aspects of the thoracolumbar spine. Such approaches have been used primarily for burst-compression fractures with significant spinal canal encroachment.[26,27]

Anterior Cervical Fusion

The anterior approach to the cervical spine is accomplished with the head fixed in tongs or pins and the neck slightly extended. The incision may be either longitudinal or transverse. A longitudinal incision is best if more than two vertebral bodies must be exposed. The anterior border of the sternocleidomastoid muscle is the major anatomical landmark for placement of the incision. The longitudinal incision follows the anterior border of this muscle, while a transverse incision is centered over the anterior border at the level of the spine to be exposed. The C5-6 level lies beneath the cricoid cartilage, C3-4 lesions lie 1 cm above the apex of the thyroid cartilage, C6-7 and C7-T1 lie approximately 1 fingerbreadth above the clavicle. Dissection through the subcutaneous tissue reveals the platysma, which is sharply divided. The platysma is then retracted to identify the medial border of the sternocleidomastoid. Blunt dissection is then accomplished between the carotid sheath laterally and the trachea and esophagus medially until the prevertebral fascia is seen. The prevertebral fascia is then incised, exposing the anterior surface of the spine and the bilaterally placed longus colli muscles. The longus colli muscles are then dissected to expose the lateral aspects of the spine. The discs are removed from the interspaces above and below the fractured vertebral body. The body can then be removed using a combination of curettes and drill, down to the level of the posterior longitudinal ligament. Fibula or rib can then be used as a strut to bridge the gap between the remaining vertebral bodies and provide for fusion (Fig. 15).

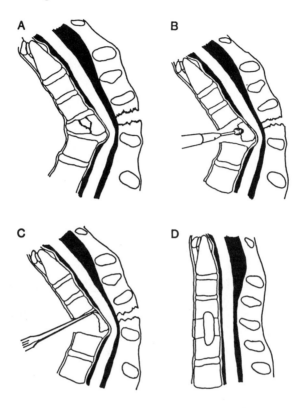

Figure 15. Significant compression fractures of cervical vertebrae often require an anterior approach (A). The fractured elements are removed with a combination of a drill (B) and curettes (C) and a bone plug or fibula strut is fashioned so as to span the distance between the two adjacent cervical vertebrae bodies (D).

Cervical immobilization for 8 to 12 weeks in a halo or cervicothoracic brace is necessary to ensure bony fusion.

Anterior Thoracolumbar Fusion

The anterolateral approach to the thoracic and upper lumbar spine requires a thoracotomy and in some cases division of the diaphragm. The midlumbar spine may be approached through a flank incision and retroperitoneal dissection. In either case, the assistance of a general or thoracic surgeon is required. Once the anterolateral aspect of the fractured vertebrae is identified, the posterior portion of the fractured vertebral body and the adjacent disc spaces are removed with an air drill and curettes. After decompressing the spinal canal, either a fibula or rib strut is used for fusion. External stabilization is maintained with a molded plastic or plaster body cast for 10 to 12 weeks.[34]

GROWTH PROBLEMS

When considering the need for cervical stabilization of spine fractures and dislocations in adolescents and children, one must always keep in mind the problems of continuing growth on the subsequent behavior of the fracture and anticipated fusion. The normal growth rate for a child slows steadily after three years of age until the growth spurt that occurs at puberty. From puberty to fourteen or fifteen years of age, the growth rate doubles. Following the acute management of these injuries, continued follow-up must be maintained until well after the growth period is over to prevent the development of spinal deformity. Spinal injuries that damage epiphyseal plates may cause an incomplete cessation of longitudinal growth or an asymmetric stimulation of epiphyseal growth resulting in scoliosis or kyphosis. Muscle imbalances secondary to the associated spinal cord injury may exacerbate this tendency. Fusing a spinal segment will effectively halt growth in this area. One series found a 91 percent incidence of spinal deformity developing six months following injury in adolescent patients. Girls under 12 years of age and boys under 14 years of age with cervical or thoracic injuries were at the greatest risk. If close follow-up is maintained and spinal deformities are detected early, proper bracing techniques may prevent further deformity. If allowed to progress untreated, severe scoliosis or kyphosis may result in death secondary to cardiopulmonary compromise (See chapter 9). Some advocate aggressive surgical intervention in children who have radiological evidence of progressive spinal deformity when the initial injuries were primarily treated nonoperatively. In a Rancho los Amigos study, 50 percent of skeletally immature patients had nonoperative therapy initially and eventually required surgical stabilization because of excessive spinal deformities. Thus, the importance of continued follow-up of children with spinal cord injuries long after the period of acute care and rehabilitation is over cannot be overemphasized.[6,14,17,19]

ANESTHETIC CONSIDERATIONS

When surgery is to be performed for spinal injuries, instability is present and careful attention must be paid to techniques of anesthetic induction, particularly intubation. The goal of intubation should be to prevent any unnecessary motion of the neck. As such, conventional endotracheal intubation is often impossible. In such cases, awake nasotracheal intubation performed blindly or under fiberoptic laryngoscopy is the preferred method of intubation. In patients with high level cervical injuries, who may have impaired diaphragmatic function and require prolonged ventilatory support, early tracheostomy should be considered. Intraoperative monitoring of the patient with spinal cord injury must be careful and include monitoring of arterial pressure as well as central venous pressure. Because of the autonomic consequences of spinal cord injury, these patients often cannot compensate for excess fluid administration or increased venous return to the heart. Thus, monitoring of the central venous pressure is often necessary. As sympathetic function of patients with spinal cord injuries above the level of T7 is unpredictable, anesthesia should be induced slowly. Autonomic excesses or deficiencies can be treated by infusion of direct vasoconstrictors (phenylephrine), vasodilators (nitroprusside or nitroglycerin), positive inotropic agents (isoproterenol), or negative inotropic agents (propranolol). Sympathetic agonists or antagonists that act directly to release catecholamines are to be avoided. In 1970, the occurrence of ventricular fibrillation after injection of succinylcholine in the spinal cord injured patient was reported. Starting with the first week and continuing over a period of six months or more, the muscle cell becomes supersensitive, and in response to a depolarizing drug such as succinylcholine, the cell membrane will depolarize and release large amounts of potassium into the circulation. This hyperkalemia may cause ventricular fibrillation and can occur up to 18 months after the original injury. Nondepolarizing relaxants such as Pavulon are effective and safe alternatives to succinylcholine.

Anesthetic Management and Emergency Care

Anesthetic risks in patients who have suffered acute spinal cord injury and must undergo emergency operations are significant. The loss of neural control and change in sympathetic reflexes can enhance the effect of anesthetic drugs, thus necessitating a careful and slow induction of anesthesia.

Preoperative assessment of these patients must be thorough and complete. Special attention should be given to injuries to other systems. Like all patients who undergo emergency surgery, patients with spinal cord injury should be considered to have a full stomach. This problem may be compounded by the loss of reflexes and abdominal tone, resulting in rapid abdominal distention. Additionally, compromised pharyngeal reflexes may increase the risk of aspiration.

Positioning can be a very difficult part of preparing these patients for surgery. In patients who are in skeletal traction and on a Stryker frame, intubation can be accomplished with the patient awake, and turning into the prone position can be achieved before anesthesia is induced. In this way the neurologic exam can be checked before the patient is asleep to ensure that no further injury has occurred. In situations in which this is not possible, extreme attention to the alignment of the spine must be maintained at all times. This requires close cooperation between the anesthesiologist and the surgeon.

Extubating patients with spinal cord injury following emergency surgery should be delayed until the patient is completely awake and can maintain a good respiratory status. After these patients have been transferred to the recovery room, they must be watched carefully for evidence of respiratory failure. It is important to remember that reasonable preoperative ventilatory function does not guarantee good postoperative respiratory function, especially if edema develops in the tissue around the vocal cords or increased edema in the spinal cord further impairs ventilatory efficiency.

Intraoperative Considerations

The following are other major intraoperative considerations that must be borne in mind constantly during the anesthetic management of children with spinal cord injury.

Cardiovascular Complications

Whenever spinal cord injury occurs at the C6 level or above, significant cardiovascular complications may result because of loss of sympathetic tone. These complications can include severe bradycardia and hyper- or hypotension. Blood pressure after such injury usually stabilizes at the level of 80 to 100 mm of mercury. This is generally adequate for perfusion of tissues when the patient is in a supine position, but it can cause significant problems if the upright position is utilized for surgery. Symptomatic hypotension occurring in such situations may require aggressive fluid resuscitation and use of vasoconstrictive agents. Normally there is no need for treatment of bradycardia in these patients, although, if it is associated with hypotension, the use of anticholinergic drugs, such as atropine, may be necessary. Electrocardiographic changes suggestive of subendocardial ischemia have been observed in patients following cord transection at the C5-6 level. In addition, there are reports of degenerative changes in the myocardium rapidly following severe injuries to the spinal cord.

Intraoperative Autonomic Hyperreflexia

Intraoperative autonomic hyperreflexia most frequently occurs when the level of anesthesia is not sufficient. Stimuli applied below the level of the lesion or bladder distension can result in paroxysmal hypertension. The usual pattern consists of initial hypertension with induction of anesthesia followed by a significant rise in blood pressure with initiation of surgery. This situation can be handled by stopping the stimulation, deepening the anesthetic level, and administering direct-acting vasoactive drugs.

Pulmonary Problems

If the patient's initial title volume is less than 3 mL/kg and the vital capacity is below 1 L, ventilatory support will be required after anesthesia and the patient should not be extubated. In general, extubation in this group of patients should be delayed until the patient is completely awake and can maintain a good respiratory status. If there is a possibility that postoperative cord edema may further compromise respiration, the endotracheal tube should be left in place.

Evoked Potential Monitoring During Surgery

The use of evoked potentials for the evaluation of disorders of the nervous system has become an important aid to the neurosurgeon and the anesthesiologist. Intraoperative monitoring of evoked potentials has become an increasingly popular procedure and is believed to aid in preserving neural function.[13,33] By repeatedly stimulating a sensory nerve in the arm or leg with an electrical shock, one can record a summated response from the scalp. Physiological characteristics of this response including the latency, amplitude, and waveform can give valuable information about the functional integrity of the anatomical pathways in the spinal cord. During manipulation of the spine and spinal cord in surgery, close attention to these potentials can provide a margin of safety. In order to gain the most benefit from this technique intraoperatively, preoperative studies should be obtained in these patients.

The amplitude of evoked potentials is so small that recording them from scalp electrodes without signal averaging is impossible. With the use of computers, these low amplitude signals can be separated from the much larger amplitude background noise composed mainly of the EEG and some nonneural electrical activity.[35] One of the most important parameters in evaluating the changes in evoked potentials is the latency of the different waveforms (Fig. 16). The latency from a peripheral nerve stimulation to the generation of an evoked potential wave component depends on many factors including the patient's body size and the position on the body of the stimulus, conduction velocity of the axons, and number of synapses in the system.[33] Nevertheless, when comparing the different tracings, which have been obtained preoperatively and at different intervals during surgery, the prolongation of latencies may indicate a pathologic process occurring as a result of surgical manipulation, such as compression of the spinal cord or traction of the axons. Since most of the fibers that transmit these poten-

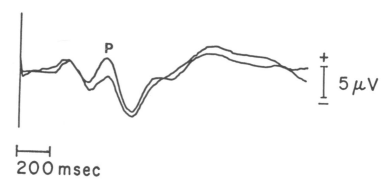

Figure 16. *Characteristic evoked potential obtained during spinal surgery. The latency of the first major positive wave (P) should remain constant throughout monitoring.*

tials are traveling through the posterior columns, localized injuries to the anterior segments of the spinal cord during surgery may not necessarily be accompanied by changes in evoked potentials.[13] This important factor should always be taken into consideration when working on the anterior segments of the spinal cord since obtaining a normal evoked potential tracing in these cases could give a false reassuring sign. The neurophysiologist, with the help of a technician who monitors these potentials, must be aware of the changes that normally occur during the operative procedure and should also be aware that various anesthetics and changes in blood pressure can affect the tracing. Use of electrocoagulation during surgery may also interfere with recording these potentials.

One of the most ominous signs of a compromise of the spinal cord during surgery is complete loss of a potential. Nevertheless, this can be the result of a technical problem, including displacement or dislodgment of an electrode. After these matters have been checked, attention should be directed to the operative site and any reversible process that includes changing the amount of retraction on the spinal cord should be attempted. Unfortunately, this is not always feasible and the changes that have occurred during surgery may be permanent. The monitoring of evoked potentials during surgery of a spinal injured patient should continue to completion of the procedure. On occasion, accumulation of epidural hematoma at the time of closure of the wound has presented with a progressive decline in amplitude and increase in latency of evoked potentials, and rapid therapeutic measures have been taken in these cases before the patient was taken from the operating room. Thus, monitoring of neural function intraoperatively using spinal evoked potentials appears to be an essential part of today's management of children with spinal cord injuries.

REFERENCES

1. Anderson JM, Schutt AH: Spinal injury in children: A review of 156 cases seen from 1950 through 1958. *Mayo Clin Proc* 55:499–504, 1980.
2. Bedbrook EB: Spinal injuries with paralysis. *Surg Neurol* 5:185–186, 1976.
3. Brodkey JS, Miller CF, Harmody RM: The syndrome of acute central cervical spinal cord injury revisited. *Surg Neurol* 14:251–257, 1980.
4. Brooks AL, Jenkins EW: Atlantoaxial arthrodesis by the wedge compression method. *J Bone Jt Surg* 60(A):279, 1978.
5. Carol M, Ducker TB, Byrnes DP: Mini-myelogram in the cervical spinal cord trauma. *Neurosurg* 7:219–229, 1980.
6. Cattell HS, Clark GL: Cervical kyphosis and instability following multiple laminectomies in children. *J Bone Jt Surg* 49(A):713, 1967.
7. Cheshire DJE: The stability of the cervical spine following the conservative treatment of fractures and fracture dislocations. *Paraplegia* 7:193–203, 1969.
8. Comarr AE: Laminectomy in patients with injuries of the spinal cord. *J Int Coll Surg* 31:437–442, 1959.
9. Comarr AE, Kaufmann AA: A survey of the neurological results of 858 spinal cord injuries. *J Neurosurg* 13:95–106, 1956.
10. Cooper PR, Cowan W: Evaluation of cervical spinal cord injuries with metrizamide myelography CT scanning. *J Neurosurg* 61:281–289, 1984.
11. Flesch JR, Leider LL, Erickson DL, et al: Harrington instrumentation and the spine. Fusion for unstable fractures and fracture dislocations of the thoracic and lumbar spine. *J Bone Jt Surg* 59(A):143, 1977.

12. Gallie WE: Fracture and dislocation of the cervical spine. *Am J Surg* 46:495, 1939.

13. Greenberg RP, Ducier TB: Evoked potentials in the clinical neuroscience. *J Neurosurg* 56:1–18, 1982.

14. Guttman L: Spinal deformities in traumatic paraplegics and tetraplegics following surgical procedures. *Paraplegia* 7:38, 1969.

15. Heiden JS, Weiss MH, Rosenberg AW, et al: Management of cervical spinal cord trauma in Southern California. *J Neurosurg* 43:732–736, 1975.

16. Holdsworth FW: Fractures, dislocations and fracture dislocations of the spine. *J Bone Jt Surg* 45(B):6–20, 1963.

17. Holmes JC, Hall JE: Fusion for instability and potential instability of the cervical spine in children and adolescents. *Orthop Clin North America* 9:923, 1978.

18. Hubbard DD: Injuries to the spine in children and adolescents. *J Bone Jt Surg* 100:56–63, 1974.

19. Kilfovle RM, Foley JJ, Norton PL: Spine and pelvic deformity in childhood and adolescence with paraplegia: A study of 104 cases. *J Bone Jt Surg* 47(A), 659, 1965.

20. Lewis J, McKibben B: The treatment of unstable fracture dislocation of the thoracolumbar spine accompanied by paraplegia. *J Bone Jt Surg* 56(B):603, 1974.

21. Morgan TH, Wharton GW, Austin GN: The results of laminectomy in patients with incomplete spinal cord injuries. *Paraplegia* 9:14–23, 1971.

22. Munro D: Treatment of fractures and dislocations of the cervical spine complicated by cervical cord and root injuries: A comparative study of fusion vs non-fusion therapy. *New Engl J Med* 264:573–582, 1961.

23. Norrell H: The treatment of unstable spinal fractures and dislocations. *Clin Surg* 125:193–208, 1978.

24. Ransohoff J, Benjamin MV, Engler G, Flamm ES: Surgical intervention in spinal cord injury in neural trauma, in Popp, AJ et al (eds): *Neural Trauma*. New York, Raven Press, 1979, pp 353–362.

25. Rogers, WA: Fractures and dislocations of the cervical spine: An end-result study. *J Bone Jt Surg* 39(A):341, 1957.

26. Rossier AD, Hussey RW, Kenzora JE: Anterior fibular interbody fusion in the treatment of cervical cord injuries. *Surg Neurol* 7:55–59, 1977.

27. Roy L, Gibson DA: Cervical spine fusion in children. *Clin Orthop* 73:146, 1970.

28. Southwick WO, Robinson RA: Surgical approaches to the vertebral bodies in the cervical and lumbar region. *J Bone Jt Surg* 39(A):364, 1957.

29. Stauffer ES, Kelly EG: Fracture dislocation of the cervical spine. *J Bone Jt Surg* 59(A):45, 1977.

30. Tator CH, Rowed DW: Current concepts in the immediate management of acute spinal cord injuries. *Can Med Assoc J* 121:1453–1464, 1979.

31. Urist M: *Clinical Orthopedics and Related Research.* J.B. Lippincott, Philadelphia, 1984, pp 46–62.
32. Wagner FC, Cherazi B: Spinal cord injury indication for operative intervention. *Surg Clin North Am* 60:1049–1054, 1980.
33. White AA, Johnson RM: Analysis of clinical stability of the cervical spine. *Clin Orthop* 109:85, 1975.
34. Whiteside TE, Ghanzanfar AS: On the management of unstable fractures of the thoracolumbar spine: Rationale for use of anterior decompression and fusion and stabilization. *Spine* 1:99, 1976.
35. Yates BJ, Thompson FJ, Mickle JP: Origin and properties of spinal cord field potentials. *Neurosurg* 11:439, 1982.

Chapter 8

Orthotic Devices
for Children

The primary goal of the immediate as well as long-term management of a child with spinal injury is to prevent further neurologic injury. The secondary goal is to promote bony healing to prevent the development of progressive spine deformity. Both goals are best accomplished by early restoration of vertebral alignment and subsequent rigid immobilization of the vertebral column either by surgical fusion or the use of an external orthotic device. Initial alignment is best achieved by various skeletal traction devices. Currently, the most popular devices are the Gardner-Wells tongs and their modifications (Fig. 1). The points of the Gardner-Wells tongs are anchored into the skull and traction can be applied in varying degrees of flexion or extension depending on the nature of the injury. In children under 18 months of age, however, the skull may not be sufficiently thick to support such tongs. For this reason, some have advocated placing burr holes and attaching wires from which traction can be utilized. However, other methods of external stabilization are presently available and may be just as adequate to achieve immediate immobilization.[9]

Orthoses are used to treat a wide variety of spinal problems ranging from minor muscle spasm to serious instabil-

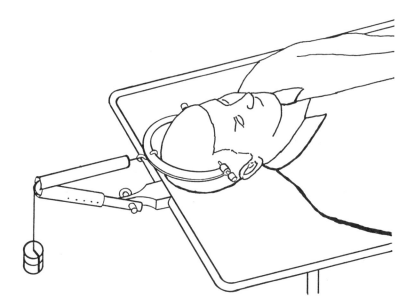

Figure 1. The Gardner-Wells tongs are currently the best device in use for maintaining skeletal traction and immobility of the cervical spine following injury. The points of the Gardner-Wells tongs can be anchored into the skull and traction applied in varying degrees of flexion or extension, depending on the nature of the injury.

ity.[1,2] The goals to be achieved determine which type of orthotic device will be utilized. The question of long-term stability of the various spinal injuries in children determines the use of either surgical fusion or external orthotic devices to maintain stability and allow healing to occur. As a general rule, if the spine injury is primarily ligamentous in nature, it is unlikely to heal in a stable fashion on a long-term basis and will most likely require surgical fusion. Bony injuries, especially in children whose growth plates or synchondroses are often affected, will heal in a stable fashion if good immobilization can be achieved.

Numerous orthotic devices are presently available to

provide external immobilization for the spine. However, special adaptations of the currently available apparatuses are often necessary to achieve satisfactory immobilization in children because of their small body size and thin skulls.

Orthoses for the cervical region may be divided into four general categories of support. The simplest is the cervical collar made from soft foam, stiff plastic, leather, or metal. The second category is that of poster braces that control the head using padded mandibular and occipital supports that are then connected by two to four rigid metal rods attached to a thoracic support. The third category is the cervical thoracic brace, which is similar to poster braces, but its thoracic support extends further down the trunk. The final and most substantial means of cervical support is provided by the halo, which provides rigid fixation of the head via pins that pierce the outer table of the skull and are attached to a metal ring. The halo ring is then connected to the trunk with longitudinal metal uprights fixed to a plastic or plaster body vest. The main means of support for the thoracic and lumbosacral spine is the body jacket, which may be made of either plastic or plaster.[2,3,4]

HISTORICAL REVIEW OF ORTHOSES

In 1852, Antoninious Mathijseu, a Flemish army surgeon, was the first to use a plaster of paris cast to immobilize a vertebral fracture. In 1887, Burrell combined traction and subsequent casting. He distracted and manipulated a cervical fracture dislocation prior to application of the cast that was designed to restrict neck motion. Halter traction was first employed in 1929 by A.F. Taylor. He stated that C5-6 hyperflexion injury was increasing because of automobile accidents. He advocated halter traction followed by immobilization in a plaster jacket for three to four weeks and then a neck brace.[1,10]

A veritable explosion of devices to exert traction on the

skull appeared in the decade prior to World War II, making it one of the major developmental periods of the treatment of cervical spinal injuries in the twentieth century. Preeminent among these was a report in 1933 by W.G. Crutchfield of a patient with a C2-3 fracture dislocation and a fractured mandible on whom halter traction could not be used. At the suggestion of Dr. C.C. Coleman, Crutchfield placed Edmonton extension tongs above both ears after a short incision and burr hole of the outer table of the skull had been made. The tongs were left in place 36 days. Crutchfield was impressed with its effectiveness and relative comfort despite the poor alignment obtained. Over the next five years, Crutchfield gained additional experience and made many modifications in the tongs until, by 1938, the Crutchfield tongs evolved as they are in use today. Crutchfield reported 43 patients treated with tongs and traction. There was only one complication, osteomyelitis. The second report by Coleman and Meredith pointed out that skeletal traction was much safer than manual reduction still much in vogue at that time.[10]

Skeletal traction devices flourished during this time. One described by Neubeiser and later modified by Selmo utilized large debarbed fish hooks that were placed under each zygoma, and then hooked to a spreader bar on which 6 to 15 lb of traction could be applied. Another method described by Hoen in 1936, consisted of two parasagittal incisions 5 cm long with burr holes at the end of each incision. After a few strokes with a Gigli saw, steel wire was passed through each of the holes that were connected to a spreader to which weight could then be applied. Also of interest was a report by Gallie in 1939 which recorded his experience with a method he had used since 1931. He used ice tongs set into the skull by a hammer blow for traction, and then applied a Minerva jacket to hold the reduction.[1,10]

In 1938, Barton first reported his tongs made specifically for skull traction, which he felt were better than others because of their supple construction, ease of installation, and low risk of skull fracture or scalp laceration. Vinke enlarged upon this principle with a more complicated but safer design. In 1953, the halo was introduced at Rancho los Amigos Hospital by Drs. Nickol, Perry, and Garrit. Its advantages included ease of application, control of rotary motion, and sound purchase on the skull. In addition, it could be used with a cast to allow ambulation of the patient while the fracture was healing.[1,10]

Contemporary trends toward early operative stabilization either posteriorly or via the anterior approach minimize the long-term use of external traction in the treatment of cervical fractures. This has resulted in the development of a number of cervical orthoses whose proper selection and application require experience with the biomechanics and physiology of the spine.

When orthotics are used to compensate for instability, a basic understanding of clinical instability is of value. It is necessary to consider which structures have been rendered nonfunctional so that appropriate support may be instituted. Spines that are unstable as a result of the loss of the functional integrity of the anterior elements are more unstable in extension. Spines unstable due to disruption to the posterior elements are more unstable on flexion. Certain orthoses protect better against anterior displacement and others protect better against posterior displacement. The clinician must be certain that it is possible to compensate for the instability with an orthotic device and that the device selected is most appropriate for the particular instability.

CATEGORIES OF ORTHOSES

Collars

The soft cervical collar is the least effective orthosis in controlling any plane of cervical motion (Fig. 2). Its main advantage is for the treatment of muscle spasms, and it serves primarily as a reminder to the child to restrict his own neck motion. The use of the soft collar in children is

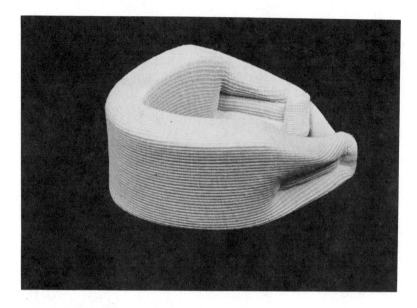

Figure 2. *The soft cervical collar is the least effective orthosis for controlling any plane of cervical motion.*

limited to those who have suffered minor neck strains and have normal radiographs. It can also be used as an adjunctive treatment after the reduction of minor degrees of atlantoaxial rotary subluxation.[4]

The stiff molded foam Philadelphia collar is significantly more effective than the soft collar in restricting cervical motion in all planes. It is considered almost as comfortable as the soft cervical collar by most patients (Fig. 3). However, the Philadelphia collar is especially weak in controlling rotation and does not provide the firm control that more rigid orthoses offer in providing cervical stability.[7]

Poster Braces

A variety of poster braces are available. The four-poster brace is considered relatively comfortable by most patients.

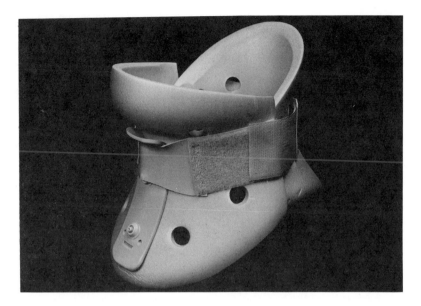

Figure 3. *The Philadelphia collar is made of stiff molded foam, is generally well tolerated by patients, and offers some degree of restriction of cervical motion in all planes.*

It ranks fourth in controlling overall motion of the neck and equals most cervicothoracic braces in controlling flexion, particularly over the middle cervical segments. Like other conventional orthoses, it is not very effective in restriction of rotation, lateral bending, and sagittal plane motion of the upper cervical spine.[4,7]

Cervicothoracic Orthoses

These orthoses are similar to the poster braces but provide greater fixation to the trunk, thus supplying greater stability. Also, these braces are more difficult to remove, which may prove quite useful for inquisitive and uncooperative young children. The most effective of these devices is the rigid cervicothoracic orthosis. This is the most effective conventional brace, but it is poor at controlling flexion at the atlantoaxial region as well as lateral bending at all levels. However, this is a relatively uncomfortable brace to wear.

A. Somi—This brace is easy to fit and can be applied with the child lying in a supine position (Fig. 4). Most children find it very comfortable to wear. Although the Somi brace does not control overall motion well, it is extremely effective in controlling flexion at the atlantoaxial and C2-3 levels and is significantly better than the more rigid cervicothoracic orthosis in this regard.[2]

B. Yale Brace—This brace was designed in an attempt to find an orthosis which was comfortable, easy to make,

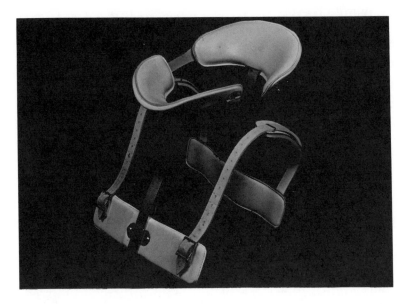

Figure 4. Four-poster braces, such as the Somi and Dennison braces, are extremely effective in controlling flexion at the upper cervical levels.

and would control cervical motion as well as the standard cervicothoracic braces. It ranks a close second to the standard cervicothoracic orthosis in controlling motion and is generally much more comfortable to wear. It shares the limitations of the other orthosis in restricting flexion and extension of only the upper part of the cervical spine. Physical therapists can make this orthosis in about one hour at a reasonable cost.[2]

Halo Apparatus

The halo brace was first introduced at the Rancho los Amigos Hospital in 1959 for the treatment of polio patients with neck problems who required stabilization. Since that time, the halo has provided a safe method of immobilizing the injured cervical spine, particularly for the restless, confused, or uncooperative patient, and has been found to be extremely useful in children as young as 17 months. The halo is generally reserved for long-term immobilization, however, the halo ring alone may be used to apply traction to achieve immediate stabilization of the spine.[3,8,11,12]

The halo consists of a stainless steel ring affixed in four opposite positions to the skull by pins that penetrate the skin and external table of the skull (Fig. 5). The pins are applied to the skull in the operating room under local anesthesia so that neurologic function can be monitored. Additional pin placement openings on the halo ring allow for alternative locations for pin placement should the pins slip, loosen, or become infected. No skin incision is necessary. The pins are introduced with a torque screwdriver and tightened to a force of 2.5 kg torque. The halo ring is attached to a horizontal frame by three or four longitudinal traction rods that can be moved to distract, flex, extend, or rotate the head within the horizontal frame. The head ring and traction rods are then stabilized by placement of sup-

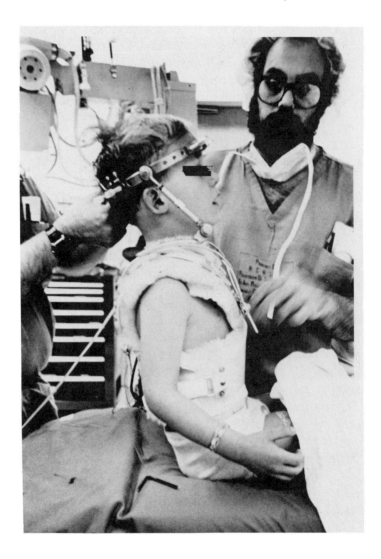

Figure 5. The halo brace is the most effective brace in controlling all motion of the cervical spine. It consists of a stainless steel ring affixed to the skull in four positions. The ring is attached through bars to a molded body jacket.

porting rods, which are incorporated into a body jacket. The body jacket can be a fitted, molded, plastic jacket or a plaster jacket. The prefabricated plastic jacket fits relatively loosely, is well padded, and is ideally suited for children with absence of sensation, such as is the situation in quadriplegics.

The halo apparatus provides complete and total fixation of the head. It allows for no rotation, lateral bending, or sagittal plane motion, including flexion and extension over the upper cervical segments. It allows almost no motion between the occiput and upper thoracic spine.

The halo has the advantage of being impossible to remove or manipulate without special wrenches. Unreliable or uncooperative children who might remove other forms of cervical orthoses will therefore be maintained in a continuous and dependable form of immobilization.

Several cautions must be kept in mind when using the halo cast for children. Children with anesthetic skin are at high risk for development of cutaneous ulcerations beneath the halo vest. The risk is particularly high if the plaster jacket is used. Also, the vest may restrict deep respiratory expansion and should not be used in children with significant respiratory problems. Similarly skin breakdown, ulceration, or infection can occur around the pin sites. Development of an epidural abscess has been reported secondary to halo placement.

In children in whom the skull is too thin to support the pins necessary for placement of the halo, and in whom other forms of braces are not satisfactory to prevent motion, the Minerva cast has been used with some success. Minerva casts can be combined with a halo ring to provide a more stable form of fixation. The Minerva cast, while providing good immobilization, is extremely uncomfortable and essentially encases the head and neck within a rigid plaster cast, which is then attached to another cast extending down over the trunk. Weight loss occurring while the cast is in place often necessitates replacement of the cast to maintain adequate immobilization.

ORTHOTIC SELECTION

Using the information based on studies determining which types of motion are best controlled by the various orthoses, these appliances may be prescribed relative to each individual clinical situation.[5] Children with Jefferson's or C1 ring fractures, if the injury is limited to the bony ring, can be satisfactorily immobilized with the Yale brace to control motion and promote healing. If the transverse ligament is also ruptured with spreading of the lateral masses, then the halo is often necessary to provide adequate stabilization. In children with dens fractures, the fracture most often occurs at the base of the dens with an associated atlantoaxial instability in all planes of motion, thus the halo is necessary to restrict this motion sufficiently to promote healing. In C2 or hangman's fractures, the maximum instability is in flexion at the second and third cervical level that is effectively controlled by the Somi brace. For the lower cervical spinal injuries, first it is necessary to determine the plane and level of primary instability. For flexion injuries at the C3 through C5 levels, the Somi brace is usually sufficient. For flexion injuries at the C5 through T1 level, the cervicothoracic brace is necessary. For extension injuries at the C3 through C5 level, either the cervicothoracic or halo braces provide stability, and for extension injuries at the C5 through T1 level, the halo cast is necessary (Fig. 6).[6,7]

By taking into account the mechanical factors as well as the clinical variables, one can select the orthosis that will most adequately protect each individual child.

	SOFT COLLAR PHILADELPHIA	CERVICOTHORACIC YALE	CERVICOTHORACIC SOMI	HALO
MUSCLE SPASMS	•			
ATLANTO-AXIAL ROTARY SUBLUXATION	•			
C1 FRACTURES WITHOUT SUBLUXATION		•	•	
WITH SUBLUXATION				•
DENS FRACTURES				•
HANGMANS FRACTURES			•	
FLEXION INJURIES C3–C5		•	•	
C5–T1		•	•	
EXTENSION INJURIES C3–C5			•	•
C5–T1				•

Figure 6. Usefulness of various orthotic devices for cervical spine problems ranging from muscle spasms to extension injuries is outlined in the chart above.

REFERENCES

1. Bunch WH, Keagy RD: *Principles of Orthotic Treatment.* New York, Mosby, 1976, pp 77–92.
2. Burger N, Lusskin R: *Atlas Orthotics.* New York, Mosby, 1975, pp 361–388.
3. Cooper PR, Maravilla KR, Skelar FH, et al: Halo immobilization of spine fractures. Indications and results. *J Neurosurg* 50: 603–610, 1979.
4. Hart DL, Johnson RM, Simmons EF, Owen J: Review of cervical orthoses. *Phys Therapy* 58: 857–860, 1978.
5. Hartman JT, Polumbo F, Hill BJ: Cineradiography of the braced normal cervical spine. *Clin Orthop Relat Res* 109: 97–101, 1975.
6. Johnson RM, Hart DL, Simmons EF, et al: Cervical orthoses, a study comparing their effectiveness in restricting cervical motion in normal subjects. *J Bone Jt Surg* 59A, 32–39, 1977.

7. Johnson RM, Owen JR, Hart DL, Callahan RA: Cervical orthoses, a guide to their selection and use. *Orthopedics* 154: 34–44, 1981.
8. Kostuik JP: Indications for the use of halo traction. *Clin Orthop Rel Res* 154: 46, 1981.
9. Kueia HA: Spinal stabilization following trauma. *Clin Orthop Rel Res* 81: 53, 1981.
10. Loeser JD: History of skeletal traction in the treatment of cervical spine injuries. *J Neurosurg* 33: 54, 1970.
11. Perry J: The halo in spinal abnormalities. Practical features and avoidance of complications. *Orthop Clin North Am* 3: 68–89, 1972.
12. Prolo GA, Runnels JB, Jamison RM: The injured cervical spine. Immediate and long-term immobilization with the halo. *JAMA* 224: 591–594, 1973.

Chapter 9

REHABILITATION OF SPINAL CORD INJURED CHILDREN

Anna J.L. Chorazy, Ann S. Valco,
Sue Cooperman, Ruth Ann Keen,
Phyllis-Ann Mandella, and Jan Titonis

Although spinal cord injury with major neurologic involvement is relatively uncommon in children, the tragedy of spinal cord injury is particularly devastating because of the many years of life that lie ahead. Until recently, it was generally accepted that all patients with spinal cord injury, regardless of age, would be subject to a premature death, usually secondary to pulmonary or renal complications. Medical advances have changed this prognosis. Based on modified life expectancy tables, DeVivo et al. estimate that a spinal cord injured male ten years of age at the time of injury will live an additional 42.2 years with complete paraplegia and an additional 28.6 years with complete quadriplegia as compared to an average of 59 years for the general population.[15]

Elsewhere in this text, the uniqueness of spinal cord injury in children is described in terms of anatomical, biomechanical, and radiological features. The wide range of developmental phenomena distinguishes the rehabilitation of spinal cord injured children and early adolescents from

that of adults. Spinal cord injured children have special
needs due to their potential for physical, intellectual,
psychological, and social growth. The developmental differences among children of varying ages and intellectual
potential must be recognized because normal development
is a template for establishing appropriate rehabilitative
goals. However, regardless of age, the level of spinal cord
injury is the most important factor in determining the
child's rehabilitative goals and long-term prognosis. The
universal goal of rehabilitative medical management of any
handicapped child is to provide the services that the child
requires to recover maximally and to compensate satisfactorily for loss or impaired function while permitting the
fullest development of physical, intellectual, psychological,
and social potential. Every effort must be made to prevent
medical complications that could interfere with rehabilitative treatment or lead to greater disability and future disease.

Children with spinal cord injury are best managed in a
rehabilitation center where expert coordinated interdisciplinary care is available. The rehabilitative medical care of
spinal cord injured children properly belongs to the physician who is knowledgeable in the care of spinal cord injury
as well as child development; for example, a highly
specialized pediatrician or pediatric physiatrist. This
physician shares responsibility and works very closely with
appropriate medical and surgical specialists and other
health-related professionals such as pediatric physiatrists,
urologists, neurologists, orthopedists, neurosurgeons, rehabilitative nurses, dietitians, physical therapists, occupational therapists, psychologists, teachers, recreational
therapists, orthotists, and social workers. When medical
findings dictate, consultation with additional specialists
may be necessary. Whenever possible, communication with
referring physicians should be maintained. A physician
coordinator may have the primary responsibility for the
coordination of all the health care services. At the Rehabili-

tation Institute of Pittsburgh, a patient-centered model is utilized. A specially trained nonphysician coordinator manages these complex cases working closely with the physician and other team members (Fig. 1).[5,59]

Optimally, rehabilitation should begin in the intensive care unit and continue in the acute care setting until the child is transferred to a comprehensive rehabilitation center. The main focus during the acute stage is on life support and the management of medical problems that, by their very nature, take priority over rehabilitation efforts. Because children are usually healthy individuals at the time of the

| | Program Coordinators | | |
	A	B	C
Medical Staff			
Dietetic Services			
Occupational Therapy			
Orthotics			
Pharmacy			
Physical Therapy			
Speech-Language Therapy			
Education			
Psychological Services			
Rehabilitation Engineering			
Rehabilitation Counseling			
Residential Living			
Social Services			
Vocational Services			
Volunteer Services			

Figure 1. The matrix model organizational chart of the Rehabilitation Institute of Pittsburgh.

accident, time spent in the acute care setting may be brief, thus facilitating transfer to a rehabilitation center sooner than adults.[18,19]

Depending upon the level of the injury, some children will also need the assistance of a respirator for all or part of the day. Aggressive efforts may be successful in weaning the patient from the respirator, however, those children who remain respirator dependent present additional problems for rehabilitation. Not all rehabilitation centers are equipped to care for such patients, but there are a few centers in the United States that are specialized and can provide such care. The acute care stay of respirator-dependent children is usually longer than for those who are not respirator dependent. The management of the respirator-dependent patient is beyond the scope of this chapter and requires the expertise of physicians and staff who specialize in the care of these patients.

Early in the course of medical management, the professional staff must help the child and the family realize that the patient will continue to grow and develop despite the devastating consequences of the injury. Life will be inexorably changed, but there are services available to help the child and the family make the necessary and painful adjustments. Depending on the severity of the spinal cord injury, a variety of medical problems result that need to be addressed in the rehabilitative process. All problems, major and minor, require appropriate diagnosis, treatment, and care.

Autonomic hyperreflexia, succinylcholine sensitivity, and pain and temperature derangements may be experienced by the child with spinal cord injury during rehabilitation. These topics are covered in detail elsewhere in this text.

BLADDER CARE

Bladder management is a major focus in the medical care of children with spinal cord injury since it is one of the determining factors for long-term survival and social acceptance. An understanding of the basic physiology of the bladder is a necessary prerequisite for a rational approach to bladder management. Normal bladder function is dependent on the integration of spinal reflexes and cortical influences. Stretching or distention of the bladder wall stimulates emptying. This is mediated through a segmental spinal reflex with the afferent arc originating with proprioreceptors in the bladder wall and ascending to the spinal cord through the pelvic nerves to the S2, S3, and S4 spinal segment levels. In the normal state, higher cortical centers inhibit the emptying reflex until the act of micturition is initiated voluntarily. The bladder then contracts by parasympathetic innervation through the pelvic splanchnic nerves. Decreased sympathetic input allows relaxation of the internal sphincter.

There are two main types of bladder dysfunction that occur as a result of spinal cord injury: the upper motor neuron (spastic or reflex bladder) and the lower motor neuron (flaccid bladder). An upper motor neuron bladder occurs when the spinal cord injury is above the T12 or conus medullaris level, leaving spinal reflexes to the bladder intact. The upper motor neuron bladder is spastic, small in capacity, and exhibits many rhythmic uninhibited contractions. However, in spite of these contractions, effective bladder emptying is not accomplished. A lower motor neuron bladder is usually seen with lesions of L1 or below in which the conus medullaris and cauda equina are damaged. There is no voluntary or reflex control of the bladder. Vesical pressure and residual urine are high. Contractions of the bladder wall are ineffective and voiding is best accomplished by increasing abdominal pressure as with the Valsalva or Crede maneuvers.

Regimens for bladder management are dependent on the age, sex, size, and weight of the child and the type of bladder. Fluid intakes and outputs are crucial in establishing programs and schedules. In babies and toddlers, for whom the use of diapers is appropriate, one still needs to assure adequate emptying of the bladder. Infants with a flaccid bladder may achieve effective emptying with Crede alone. However, Crede should never be used if there is any suspicion of vesico-ureteral reflex. Once the child reaches school age, diapers are no longer appropriate and their continued use may be detrimental to the child's self-esteem and self-image. Clean, intermittent catheterization (CIC) is an alternative and can be instituted at any age.[34,52]

The goal of CIC is not only to empty the bladder, but also to prevent infection and retrain the bladder. In most cases, a catheter-free bladder with low residual and sterile urine should be achievable over a three- to six-month period. The CIC technique is relatively simple and can be taught to parents and patients. Children as young as five years of age can master this technique of self-catheterization. Initially, depending on the child's fluid intake, it is generally necessary to perform CIC every four hours. As residual urinary volumes decrease and the volume voided spontaneously or obtained by Crede increases, the time interval between catheterizations can be lengthened to six to eight hours. In between the CIC, the patient should attempt to void spontaneously or with stimulation, such as Crede, maintaining at least a four-hour bladder emptying schedule. As the bladder progressively empties more completely, the time interval for CIC may be decreased to twice or even once a day. Children with quadriplegia will need detailed assistance with CIC. Also, very young children may be unable to independently perform the maneuvers necessary for CIC.[1,10,28,54]

Medications may be a necessary adjunct to the bladder training program. Bethanecol chloride (Urecholine) a parasympathomimetic drug may be used to help the bladder contract. Phenoxybenzamine hydrochloride (Dibenzyline), an alpha-adrenergic blocking agent, may be used to decrease sphincter resistance. Oxybutynin chloride (Ditropan) and propantheline bromide (Pro-Banthine), anticholinergic drugs, may be used to inhibit bladder spasms. Imipramine hydrochloride (Tofranil), an antidepressant with anticholinergic properties, may be beneficial in decreasing the spontaneous emptying of the bladder.

Avoidance of repeated urinary tract infection and overdistention of the bladder are paramount in maintaining normal bladder and renal function. The Foley catheter should be removed as soon as possible and bladder retraining started. If infection occurs, it should be treated aggressively. Urinary asepsis may be helped by acidification of the urine with oral vitamin C, and urinary antiseptic agents such as methenamine mandelate and hippuric acid.[43] Urolithiasis is a potential complication of persistent urinary tract infection. This is more common in children than in adults and should be looked for if the urine cannot be kept free of infection.[21,64] It is recommended that an intravenous pyelogram (IVP) be performed in the acute phase following spinal cord injury to establish a baseline and rule out any abnormalities. The IVP should be repeated at yearly intervals or more frequently if necessary. Other bladder studies such as cystoscopy, cystometrogram, and renal scan may be obtained as clinically indicated. Weekly urinalysis, regular urine cultures, and blood urea nitrogen and creatinine levels should be obtained for monitoring during bladder retraining programs.[64]

BOWEL REGULATION

Bowel control is a major problem for children with spinal cord injury. Fecal soiling is embarrassing and socially unacceptable. Inadequate elimination of fecal material may result in nausea, vomiting, poor appetite, listlessness, and increased incidence of urinary tract infection secondary to partial ureteral obstruction.

An understanding of the basic physiology of the bowel is a necessary prerequisite for a rational approach to bowel management. Distention of the rectum is the usual stimulus for defecation. The motor innervation of the rectum and internal and external sphincters is through the sacral nerves S2, S3, and S4. The striated external sphincter is dependent on its extrinsic nerve supply for its tone. The internal sphincter can function separately from its nerve supply and responds to stimulation of the autonomic nervous system. Distention of the rectum causes relaxation of the internal sphincter and a descent of fecal material. If the nervous control is intact, the external sphincter, which is under voluntary control, then contracts and holds the feces within the rectum. The urge to defecate is then recognized in the brain. Here, it is either acted on or suppressed. In the spinal cord injured patient, depending on the type and level of lesion, the external sphincter may not be able to contract effectively or, if it does, for only a limited period of time.

The goal of bowel training is effective controlled emptying of the large intestine. This is usually accomplished by a combination of dietary management, stool softeners, and some form of rectal stimulation. Dietary management includes the establishment of regular eating patterns and the consumption of a well-balanced diet with the appropriate amounts of fluids and fiber. Fiber can be increased by eating bran, fresh and dried fruits, fresh vegetables, whole grain products, and nuts.

It may be necessary to add a stool softener with or without a bowel stimulant. There are many commercial preparations on the market that are useful and effective in adolescents. However, in small children, the dose and the mode of delivery may not be satisfactory. We have found that a combination of the stool softener, blond psyllium seed coatings (Siblin) mixed with pureed prunes (lekvar) is most effective and acceptable. Mineral oil is contraindicated for routine use because it depletes the body of fat soluble vitamins and its use often results in rectal seepage. Rectal stimulation in the form of digital stimulation may be effective. However, it should be stressed that whatever form of rectal stimulation is used, regular timing is necessary in order to achieve retraining. If digital stimulation is not sufficient, one may proceed to a more effective method such as the use of suppositories. It is best to start out with the mildest type, such as glycerine suppositories, and progress to a more stimulating agent such as bisacodyl suppositories, if necessary. Suppositories should be inserted on a regular schedule and parents should be instructed on their proper insertion so that they will be effective. Initially, the suppository can be used on a daily basis and then decreased to an alternate-day program. Daily defecation is not a necessity. Enemas usually are avoided because of the potential problems of fluid and electrolyte absorption through the gut and the rare possibility of eliciting autonomic hyperreflexia. Enemas may cause fluid and electrolyte imbalances, especially in the very young child with small fluid compartments. A special disadvantage to an enema program is that enemas do not lend themselves to independent self-administration.

The usual bowel regimen for a young child emphasizes not only a well-balanced diet, adequate fluids, use of manual stimulation, liberal use of stool softeners, and, when appropriate, suppositories, but also a regular toileting time. The child should be placed on the commode at the same time on a daily basis. The best time to capitalize physiologically on the gastrocolic reflex is approximately a half hour after a major meal. The child needs to feel comfortable and relaxed. Therefore, appropriate seating with truncal support and feet supported on the floor or raised platform is optimal. There are many specialized commode chairs available that have these features, or home commodes may be adapted inexpensively. It is not uncommon that the patient can evacuate by sitting on the commode at regular intervals after bowel retraining has become established. For well-motivated older children with lesions of L2 or lower, biofeedback training may provide an alternative and more acceptable method of bowel retraining.[68]

An ineffective bowel program can present in many ways. One must be alert to the subtle signs such as loss of appetite, abdominal distention, and general malaise. The more overt signs such as vomiting, abdominal pain, or cramping and diarrhea are less easily missed. It is important to differentiate true diarrhea from impaction. The diarrhea of obstruction is due to seepage around an impaction of stool and usually is accompanied by other signs that may have been overlooked. The child need not appear acutely ill. In the typical gastrointestinal viral or bacterial infection, the child may have fever and more frequent and explosive symptoms. When in doubt, an impaction can always be ruled out by a simple rectal examination.

SKIN CARE

Skin problems resulting from prolonged pressure can lead to serious complications for the child with cord injury. Prevention must be emphasized from the beginning as the best treatment of pressure sores or decubiti. Prevention is best accomplished by frequent position changes to avoid prolonged pressure, especially over bony prominences. The most common sites for the development of decubiti are the ischial, sacral, malleolar, trochanteric, and coccygeal prominences.[27] Position change should be done at least every two hours when the child is in bed or as often as every ten to fifteen minutes when sitting in a chair. No cushion or mattress, no matter how well designed, obviates the necessity of frequent position changes and careful skin checks. All children need to be given frequent reminders in order for them to incorporate this into their habit behavior. Children must be taught to monitor their own skin as to moisture, color, irritation, and breakdown. A small area of superficial redness can mask a larger, deeper triangular area of necrosis beneath. Children as young as five years of age can be taught the necessity and mechanics of skin monitoring. Young children are often more compliant in caring for their skin than adolescents.

Patients and their parents must be made aware that there are several classic ways decubiti develop, including friction, shearing, rubbing forces, pressure, heat, and extreme cold. These mechanisms should be kept in mind at all times, but especially during dressing, transferring, or any change of position.[2] Moisture secondary to urinary incontinence can also predispose to skin breakdown. Frequent changes of clothing or diapers may be necessary. Improperly fitted braces and casts often predispose the child to pressure sores. All casts should be properly and sufficiently padded prior to application. Parents also need be advised about the possibility of frostbite or sunburn when the patient is outdoors in very cold or sunny, hot weather, since these children do not have the protection of appreciating extremes of heat or cold.[11]

One of the major goals of rehabilitation of the child with spinal cord injury is the establishment of sitting tolerance. A graduated sitting program using a reclining wheelchair is helpful in preventing decubiti. Specialized cushions, which aid the child in maintaining a seated position for a long period of time, are available.[60] In our experience, the two-inch T-foam cushion is most utilitarian for children with paraplegia and for some children with quadriplegia in terms of ease of transfer, lightness, cost, and general maintenance. Gel cushions, although useful for some patients, may be too heavy for others to easily lift. There are specialized transducers available to help train children to monitor pressure relief.[25]

There also are a variety of mattresses available, such as sheepskin, water mattresses, and alternating air mattresses. Most of these specialized cushions and mattresses are expensive. Often an inexpensive egg crate mattress or cushion is sufficient. For those children with severe or multiple decubiti, a clinitron bed may be necessary to relieve pressure temporarily to promote healing.

If skin redness does occur, the first and most important step is the avoidance of pressure over the area. If it is mild, pressure relief alone may be sufficient to minimize progression and achieve healing. If there is any evidence of skin breakdown, additional measures may be necessary, such as the application of a protective, semipermeable membrane, such as Opsite®, or other synthetic protective products. All pressure areas must be kept clean and dry. If the decubitus is deeper or appears inflamed, a variety of topical agents may be indicated. Occasionally, povidone-iodine (Betadine) and hydrogen peroxide cleansing, as well as wet-to-dry dressings with dilute acidic acid or saline, may be helpful. If the decubitus is more severe with eschar formation, debridement either by topical enzymes or surgery may be necessary.

There is a known relationship between the adequacy of the child's nutritional status and a predisposition for the development of pressure sores and the ability to heal rapidly once a decubitus develops. Therefore, an adequate protein diet plus supplements of vitamins A and C, folic acid, and mineral supplements of iron and zinc are mandatory for the maintenance of healthy skin integrity.[29]

NUTRITION

The nutritional management of a child with spinal cord injury involves consideration of not only metabolic and physical changes caused by the trauma, but also the proper nutrition needed for growth and development. The first step in developing a nutritional care plan is a comprehensive assessment (Table 1).

In order to achieve an anabolic state, protein requirements may be twice the Recommended Dietary Allowances.[22,50] This protein should be provided in a palatable high biologic form such as meats, poultry, fish, and nuts.[49] Sufficient calories also must be provided. Using cream instead of milk in cooking and on cereal, adding extra butter and sugar to certain foods, using mayonnaise, gravy and

---

Table I

Components of a Nutritional Assessment for Spinal Cord Injured Children and Adolescents*

A. Food Habits
   1. Typical day's intake prior to injury
   2. Vitamin and mineral supplements
   3. Appetite prior to injury and present time
   4. Favorite foods
   5. Disliked foods
   6. Time(s) of the day patient presently appears most hungry
   7. Food allergies
B. Physical Problems Related to Food and Fluids
   1. Ability to chew and swallow
   2. Constipation or diarrhea
   3. Bladder function
C. Biochemical Findings
   1. Potassium
   2. Sodium
   3. Albumin
   4. BUN
   5. CBC
   5. Total protein
D. Clinical Findings
   1. Weight to height (use National Center for Health Statistics [NCHS] growth charts)
   2. Skin integrity, elasticity
   3. Musculature vs. subcutaneous fat
   4. Attitude/behavior

---

*Obtained from family and/or patient and/or hospital records.

bacon bits, all provide extra calories with little increase in the volume of food eaten. Commercial preparations such as glucose polymers, fatty emulsions, and high calorie, high protein drinks may be of value for some children. Many children are able to meet their nutritional requirements on a prescribed diet, however, it may be necessary to enlist parents' assistance in getting the child to consume sufficient nutrients. Families tend to focus a lot of energy on their children's food intake during the beginning stages of rehabilitation and they are eager to assist in this endeavor.

They are encouraged to help at mealtime and bring in the child's favorite foods.

Alterations in digestion and gastric and duodenal ulcers occasionally occur. They can be managed effectively with medication such as cimetidine (Tagamet) and antacids. Caffeine, cola, chocolate, pepper, and chili and curry powders should be eliminated until such ulcers are healed.

Dietary modifications are indicated for hypo- or hyperkalemia and hypo- and hypernatremia. Potassium rich foods include bananas, baked potatoes, and prune, orange and tomato juices. Sodium intake may need to be restricted with the exclusion of table salt, salted or smoked meats, including luncheon meats, bacon, sausage and hotdogs, highly salted foods, catsup, olives, soysauce, cheese, and peanut butter.

When a child has achieved a stabilized anabolic state, caloric modifications may be necessary to prevent obesity. It has been our practice to establish a basal metabolic rate and add 10 percent to 30 percent for activity (crutch walking requires two to four times the energy expenditure as walking for a normal child, wheelchair ambulation requires the same energy expediture as walking for a normal child). The reduction of 500 calories per day will result in a one pound weight loss per week.[46] Due to the paralysis and subsequent muscle loss, the child with spinal cord injury should be maintained at or slightly below his/her ideal weight for height. Care should be taken to provide sufficient calories and nutrients for growth without causing obesity.[13,29]

INFECTION SURVEILLANCE

Evaluation of infection in a child with spinal cord injury is complicated by the child's lack of sensation to pain, as well as impaired temperature control. The quadriplegic child, in particular, may manifest a transient modest elevation of body temperature in response to environmental heat.

However, persistent fever is due to either viral or bacterial infection, and careful determination of the site and type of infection is important.

Children with spinal cord injury are as prone as all children to the usual respiratory infections and diseases of childhood, with viral illnesses being more common than those caused by bacteria. The most common sites of viral infections are the upper respiratory tract and pharynx. Antibiotics are not helpful in viral illnesses. Bacterial infections commonly occur in the middle ear, lungs, urinary tract, and skin. Cultures of throat and urine should be routine in children with significant fever in order to determine the cause of infection.

Children with spinal cord injury have a significant predisposition to urinary tract infections. Infections by gram-negative organisms may lead to sepsis and gram-negative shock if not recognized and treated promptly. Therefore, blood cultures are also necessary if urinary tract infection is suspected and the child appears clinically ill. The classic symptoms of dysuria and abdominal pain may not be appreciated by the patient. Orchitis may present a problem in males and should be considered as a cause for infection.

Children with cervical and high thoracic cord lesions have the additional problem of decreased ability to cough and clear secretions. Because of the potential for lower respiratory problems, these patients need to be mobilized as early as possible and taught to do periodic manual coughing, deep breathing, glossopharyngeal breathing techniques, and pulmonary training in order to prevent complications of pulmonary atelectasis and pneumonia. When such children develop upper respiratory infections, they may need the added assistance of such measures as chest physical therapy and postural drainage to prevent potentially fatal complications.

Skin infection that may be secondary to a pressure sore or ingrown toenail may begin as a minor problem, but must be assessed accurately. If neglected, they can lead to more serious infections. An overlooked infected ingrown toenail may be the precipitating factor for autonomic hyperreflexia in patients with quadriplegia.[20]

Immobility predisposes patients to poor circulation and venous stasis, thereby increasing susceptibility to thrombophlebitis. Antiembolic elastic stockings and early mobilization help to prevent this complication. Children are less affected by this complication than adults. In spite of the rarity of thrombophlebitis in children it must be considered when evaluating a patient with fever. Serial measurement of the lower extremities assist in diagnosing this problem. Occasionally, more sophisticated diagnostic studies, such as plethysmography and Doppler studies are needed to make this diagnosis. Short-term anticoagulation may be used initially, but is not indicated on a long-term basis.[46]

HYPERCALCEMIA

Hypercalcemia and bone demineralization frequently occur in rapidly growing children and adolescents following spinal cord injury or other disorders that result in enforced immobilization.[14,56] However, significant hypercalcemia, even during the first four to eight weeks following injury, is rare.[61] According to Maynard, hypercalcemia is probably secondary to an imbalance of osteoblastic and osteoclastic activity.[42] Bone resorption is increased and the high calcium load is inadequately excreted by the kidney because of the calcium's direct effect on the kidney tubules. In their retrospective study of youths with spinal cord injury, Nand and Goldschmidt reported a 19.8 percent incidence of hypercalcemia as defined by a calcium level of greater than 10.6 mg percent.[48] Tori and Hill reported a 23.6 percent incidence of hypercalcemia with levels in excess of 11.6 mg percent. The highest calcium levels were recorded between 1 and 12 weeks postinjury and did not always correlate with the severity of the paralysis. These elevated levels usually were temporary, returning to normal within three to four months without specific therapy.[63]

Clinically, hypercalcemia may present with symptoms of abdominal pain and discomfort, anorexia, nausea, vomiting, malaise, headache, polydipsia, polyuria, or lethargy. Early mobilization and weight bearing on a tilt table aid in normalizing the elevated calcium level. It is not necessary to limit dietary calcium intake. If hypercalcemia persists after mobilization, a diet of less than 400 mg of calcium per day for several weeks may be indicated.[23]

HETEROTOPIC OSSIFICATION

Heterotopic ossification, the abnormal deposition of bone in tissue occurs in both neurologic and orthopedic disorders. Venier and Ditunno reported incidences of 16 percent to 53 percent of heterotopic bone formation in patients of all ages with spinal cord injury. The hips are the most common area of involvement, followed by the knees, elbows, and shoulders. Heterotopic ossification usually manifests itself one to four months postinjury, but it takes 18 to 24 months for heterotopic bone to mature from the initial abnormal calcium deposition. The extent of ossification may range from an incidental finding on x-ray films, to very extensive involvement that limits the range of motion of the joint and may cause severe ankylosis.[67]

Heterotopic ossification may present clinically in a variety of forms. Subtle signs initially may be confused with a fracture or an abscess because the inflammatory reaction of increased redness, warmth, and swelling is present in all three cases. The patient may present with a gradual loss of motion of the joint involved. A high index of suspicion is needed to make this diagnosis early, especially in children. Three-phase bone scans are often positive four to six weeks prior to evidence of ossification on x-ray films.[9]

Treatment involves physical therapy with active range

of motion, good positioning, and splinting. Surgery is contraindicated in the early stages because the process will continue to progress as the bone matures. Even after the heterotopic bone matures, which takes approximately two years, there is still some question of the value of surgery since the bone may recur. Etidronate disodium is recommended and used for the prevention of heterotopic bone in adults, but it is not 100 percent effective and has some unpleasant side effects. Since this drug prevents mineralization of bone, it is not recommended for use in growing children.[62]

SCOLIOSIS

Scoliosis, a lateral rotary curvature of the spine; lordosis, an abnormally increased curvature of the lumbar spine; and kyphosis, an abnormally increased posterior curvature of the thoracic spine are frequently seen in children who have sustained a spinal cord injury. Banniza et al. reported a 65 percent incidence of scoliosis greater than 15° in children under the age of 15 with paraplegia.[4] Mayfield reported that of 40 patients between the ages of 0 and 18 years, 96 percent developed spinal curvatures.[39] Of these patients, 92 percent developed scoliosis and 62 percent showed excessive lumbar lordosis. The most significant factor in the development of scoliosis is the age of the child at the time of the injury. The younger the child at the time of the injury, the greater the potential for spinal curvature.[3,35,57]

Spinal curvature is secondary to asymmetric or unequal muscle pull on the vertebral structures and may progress rapidly during periods of growth. Children with lesions of T12 or lower are less likely to develop these complications because the abdominal, back, and vertebral musculature is fully innervated. There is some disagreement as to the effects of laminectomy and fusion on the development of spinal curvature.[37,39]

As the scoliosis progresses in severity, gravitational forces and the unequal muscle pull may cause the pelvis to deviate from its perpendicular position resulting in pelvic obliquity. The functional implication of pelvic obliquity may include unequal ischial weight bearing in sitting, apparent leg length discrepancy, and disturbance in sitting balance. As the pelvis is pulled from its perpendicular position, the body weight becomes concentrated on one ischium, predisposing this area to skin breakdown.

If scoliosis is allowed to progress without intervention and the curvature exceeds 60°, cardiopulmonary function may be compromised. As the degree of the curve increases, the rotary deformity of the vertebrae and rib cage also increases.[33] This causes a decrease in the size of the chest cavity, resulting in limitation of lung expansion. In extremely severe scoliosis, intestinal and bladder function may also be affected.[4]

Although the development of spinal curvature cannot be prevented in the young child with spinal cord injury, there are a variety of treatment measures most effectively used in combination that may delay its onset and slow its progression. These include the following:

1. Good bed positioning, including frequent turning and strategic use of pillows.
2. Wheelchair inserts, including truncal supports.
3. Bracing, including supportive jackets and thoraco-lumbosacral orthoses.
4. Exercises to maintain spinal mobility.

Because scoliosis is extremely complex and difficult to control, early detection and intervention are vital to maintain passive spinal mobility until maturation of the spinal skeleton has occurred. The status of the spinal curvature should be monitored on a regular bases with x-ray examination for comparative measurements. These conservative measurements are often not sufficient to maintain adequate spinal alignment and surgery may be necessary. Mayfield reported that in his review of 49 patients under the age of 18, 61 percent of the juvenile patients and 33 percent of the adolescent patients required spinal fusion for progressive scoliosis.[39]

SPASTICITY

Spasticity is commonly seen in patients with spinal cord injury and usually presents within a few weeks to months following the injury. It is the hyperexcitability of the stretch reflex that is clinically manifested by hyperactive deep tendon reflexes, clonus, and a velocity-dependent resistance to movement. Spasticity is more severe with incomplete than complete lesions, but is rarely seen in cauda equina injuries.

Spasticity may appear initially as flexor spasms. Ultimately, however, the extensor component usually becomes dominant. Although the increased tone accompanying spasticity may provide needed support for activities of daily living or transfer activities, more commonly it interferes with functioning and contributes to the development of contractures.

Spasticity may be partially moderated by good positioning and splinting, early weight bearing, and an appropriate exercise program. A rapid rise in spasticity may occur with irritant stimuli, such as tight clothing, decubiti, ingrown toenails, heterotopic bone formation, and urinary tract infection. Spasticity will return to its previous level following the remediation of these problems.

The decision to use pharmaceutical intervention for spasticity should be made by the physician, but should include input from members of the rehabilitation team because the medications used in treating spasticity may reduce function by taking away useful muscle tone. The drugs used most often for spasticity are baclofen (Lioresal), diazepam (Valium), and dantrolene sodium (Dantrium).[70,71] Each of these medications has specific advantages and disadvantages, and all have a very narrow margin between therapeutic effectiveness and unacceptable side effects when used with small children. Baclofen is not recommended for children under 12 years of age but is probably the best choice for older patients since it acts primarily at the spinal cord level and is less likely to reduce voluntary motor control. However, it may cause transient drowsiness or hallucinations or lower the seizure threshold, especially if the dosage is raised or lowered too quickly. Diazepam is often preferred in children because it can be given in small doses with effective control of the spasticity. It may cause drowsiness but usually not to an incapacitating degree. The third major antispasmodic, dantrolene sodium, works at the level of the muscle. Its primary side effect is liver damage, which is more common in adult women than in children. However, all patients on dantrolene sodium should have periodic liver function studies.

GENERAL HEALTH CARE MAINTENANCE

Spinal cord injured children must receive expert care for their unique problems that result from their injury, but should not be neglected in terms of periodic comprehensive general health care assessment and preventive maintenance. All children should have routine screening of their overall health status with monitoring of growth and development, dentition, nutrition, blood pressure, and immunization status. All children should receive the basic diphtheria, pertussis, tetanus, and polio vaccines with appropriate boosters as well as measles, mumps, and rubella vaccines. Children with high spinal cord injuries and severe kyphoscoliosis who are prone to frequent respiratory infections should receive a yearly influenza vaccine as well as pneumococcal vaccine.[55]

PRINCIPLES OF REHABILITATION

Rehabilitation goals for the pediatric patient with spinal cord injury are basically the same as those for adult patients, i.e., the development of body management skills and the maximization of independence. However, the treatment program for the pediatric patient must be guided by certain principles of normal development:

1. body proportions change during maturation;
2. motor skills are refined as the neurologic system matures;
3. learning occurs through play;
4. children require unstructured time;
5. children progress from dependence to independence;
6. children are part of a family system;
7. children need both discipline and rewards.

As children develop physically, the relative proportion of the limbs to the trunk changes. These changes not only affect motor abilities but also the location of the center of gravity. These factors become significant when children with spinal cord injury must use their arms to support their trunk and legs. For example, a young child whose arms are proportionately shorter than his trunk may find climbing stairs with long leg braces impossible.

Motor skills develop and become refined as children grow and integrate their newly acquired abilities into their motor repertoire. For example, young children first develop bilateral upper extremity coordination and then refine that ability to coordinate ipsilateral function. Therefore, a very young child may be able to propel a wheelchair forward and backward, but may not have sufficient upper extremity coordination to negotiate turns.

Children learn through play. This premise suggests that treatment objectives are most often accomplished through games rather than through strict exercise regimens. For a young child working on strengthening upper extremity skills, prone scootering may be more effective than lifting weights. Prone scootering is an age-appropriate exploratory activity that also incorporates upper extremity strengthening, endurance and coordination. Since scootering is an enjoyable activity, young children may be more likely to engage in it voluntarily.

Periods of unstructured time are important for everyone, particularly for children and adolescents with spinal cord injury who are adjusting to a major loss and may have many demands placed on them. These periods provide an opportunity for the young patient to be alone or with others as an individual rather than as a patient with physical disabilities. Children should have interludes from their hectic schedules to engage in solitary play, watch television, or talk with friends.

As a child's physical, cognitive, and emotional skills develop, they become progressively more independent. Treatment and family expectations must be guided by age-appropriate developmental skills and physical abilities. For instance, a two-year-old child with paraplegia may have the physical capacities to put shoes on, but this activity usually is not learned until a later age after other skills have been mastered.

The child is an important member of the family unit and the family must be considered as an integral part of the treatment process. Treatment rationale, expectations, and techniques should be shared with the family so that the family members understand, support, and participate in the program. Family needs may include variations in the treatment program. For example, outdoor mobility and adapted fishing equipment may be important treatment objectives for the adolescent whose family frequently enjoys fishing trips.

Children and adolescents with spinal cord injury require both discipline and praise as do all young people, but their application should be tempered by an understanding of the many and, at times, frustrating demands placed on these children. Children with spinal cord injury must be helped to realize that unacceptable behavior remains unacceptable in spite of their physical disability.[66]

The following series of charts outlines the rehabilitation goals in children with various levels of spinal cord injury (Table II). (Text continues page 222.)

Table II
Comprehensive Rehabilitation Program
for Children with Spinal Cord Injury

LEVEL AND FUNCTION REMAINING	TREATMENT GUIDELINES	FUNCTIONAL OBJECTIVE	FUNCTIONAL EQUIPMENT
C₄ respiration scapular elevation neck movements (SCM)	—passive range of motion	tolerance for upright position	—tilt table, manual or electric
	—improve head control and strengthen remaining neck and shoulder musculature		—reclining wheelchair with cushion, elevating leg rests and trunkal supports
	—establish variety of positioning alternatives to prevent contractures, reduce spasticity, prevent pressure areas	safe bathing	—sling in bathtub or reclining shower chair
	—may require respiratory program including bronchial drainage, manual cough, diaphragm strengthening, change of position every two hours. A corset may be used to increase abdominal support.	self-feeding usually not energy-efficient even with devices	—cup with long straw, if placed appropriately, facilitates independent drinking
		control of environment including lights, TV, radio, telephone	—touch-access environmental controls unit
			—automatic dial telephone
	—increase tolerance for upright position by increasing angle of and length of time on tilt table and in wheelchair (use cushion in chair to prevent pressure areas)	electric wheelchair propulsion	—touch-access system, mouthstick or sip 'n puff control
			—electric wheelchair
	—train in use of adaptive equipment	typing (about 5 words/min)	—mouthstick or touch-access electric typewriter with power return button, self-correcting ribbon or other correcting mechanism, roll of paper
	—explore alternatives for prevocational training		

C4

—patient and family training in physical care, functional activities, use and maintenance of all equipment
—provide home program

return to school (adapted or special school placement may be necessary)

—angled tray or work surface
—adapted electric typewriter
—adapted tape recorder for note taking
—electric page turner for reading
—adapted computer

C5
shoulder elevation
shoulder abduction (partial)
scapular rotation and adduction
elbow flexion (partial)

—passive range of motion
Note: less than normal range is desirable in the finger flexors (for tenodesis grasp) and the back extensors (for sitting stability)
—strengthen all remaining musculature
—establish positioning alternatives (see C4)
—teach compensatory body management skills
—may require respiratory program (see C4)
—increase tolerance for upright position (see C4)
—teach assisted pressure relief techniques
—train in use of adaptive equipment
—explore alternatives for prevocational/vocational training
—patient and family training in physical care, functional activities, use and maintenance of all equipment
—provide home program

self-feeding (may not be energy-efficient for some patients)

assist with hygiene (may not be energy efficient for some patients)

other—see functional objectives listed under C4

—mobile arm support, ball bearing feeder, or bedside slings
—dynamic tenodesis splint, externally powered flexor hand splint, or universal cuff
—special feeding equipment may include: scoop dish or plate with plate guard, nonslip surface such as Dycem, nontip cup or long straw, built-up handles on silverware
—splints and equipment listed above
—electric razor
—electric toothbrush
—equipment remains as stated in C4 but objectives are accomplished more efficiently

Table II cont.

LEVEL AND FUNCTION REMAINING	TREATMENT GUIDELINES	FUNCTIONAL OBJECTIVE	FUNCTIONAL EQUIPMENT
C6 shoulder flexion and extension elbow flexion supination wrist extension weak sensory function in hand	—passive range of motion (teach self-range as indicated) *Note:* less than normal range is desirable in the finger flexors and back extensors. Greater than normal range is desirable in the hamstrings (for lower extremity dressing). Full range is desirable in elbow extension (for locking elbows for pressure relief and transfers). —strengthen remaining musculature —may require respiratory program (see C4) and strengthening of accessory breathing musculature —establish positioning alternatives (see C4) —increase tolerance to upright position (see C4) —teach pressure relief techniques including wheelchair pushups and use of cushion —teach compensatory body management skills —teach activities of daily living (ADLs) including hygiene, dressing, feeding, bathing, skin care, and transfers	relieve ischial pressure in wheelchair self-feeding assist with dressing assist with hygiene	—arms of wheelchair used for sitting pushups —wheelchair cushion —universal cuff —special feeding equipment including scoop dish or plate guard, nonslip surface such as Dycem, quad-cup, rocker knife, spork, utensils with built-up handles —dynamic tenodesis splint (when pinch is necessary) —button hook —velcro closures —pant loops, zipper pull, and other adaptations —velcro closure shoes —electric razor —electric toothbrush —toileting devices including adaptations for catheter and leg bag, and suppository inserter —mirror on gooseneck for skin inspection

—train in use of adaptive equipment	assisted/independent transfers	—sliding board —loops or trapeze for bed mobility —grab bars
—explore alternatives for prevocational/vocational training	wheelchair propulsion	—electric or manual wheelchair with rim projections —brake extensions
—patient and family training in physical care, functional activities, use and maintenance of all equipment	tolerance for upright position	—tilt table (manual or electric) —reclining wheelchair with cushion, elevating leg rests and trunkal supports *Note:* once tolerance for the upright position is achieved, standard wheelchair may be substituted for reclining wheelchair
—provide home program	self-bathing (may be independent except for transfers)	—tub seat or shower chair —hand-held spray attachment —bath mitt with pocket for soap
	writing	—dynamic tenodesis splint —pen/pencil holding device —pencil or dowel in universal cuff or interlaced between fingers
	typing (about 20 words per minute)	—electric typewriter with automatic return
	using a telephone	—touch-tone telephone —pencil or dowel held in universal cuff or laced between fingers for dial telephone —automatic dial telephone
	return to school (can be mainstreamed)	—electric typewriter —writing devices —adapted tape recorder for note taking

Table II cont.

LEVEL AND FUNCTION REMAINING	TREATMENT GUIDELINES	FUNCTIONAL OBJECTIVE	FUNCTIONAL EQUIPMENT
C_6		driving a car (may be independent for some patients)	—wheelchair bag for carrying supplies —computer —angled tray or work surface —hand controls —shoulder harness —driving knob or cuff
C_7 partial grasp and release (gross) weak shoulder depression active elbow extension sensory function of hand	—passive range of motion (teach self-range as indicated) *Note:* see passive range C_6. —strengthen remaining musculature —may require respiratory program and strengthening of accessory breathing musculature —establish positioning alternatives with increased emphasis on sitting and standing —teach compensatory body management skills —teach pressure relief techniques including wheelchair pushups and use of cushion —teach ADLs including hygiene, dressing, feeding, bathing, skin care, transfers, and homemaking skills	relieve ischial pressure in wheelchair independent self-feeding independent dressing (except for shoes) assist with hygiene independent transfers independent wheelchair propulsion	—arms of wheelchair used for sitting pushups —wheelchair cushions —utensils with built-up handle —weave fork in fingers —universal cuff —button hook or velcro closures —zipper pulls —pant loops —sock aid —see C_6 —more energy-efficient —hairbrush with large handle —grab bars in bathroom, bedroom as needed —sliding board —rim projections if desired

C7

	tolerance for upright position	—tilt table—manual or electric —reclining wheelchair with cushion, elevating leg rests and trunkal supports *Note*: see C_6
—ambulation training for the younger patient (short distances only) —train for wheelchair mobility in the community —train in use of adaptive equipment —explore alternatives for prevocational/vocational training —patient and family training in physical care, functional activities, use and maintenance of all equipment —provide home program	assisted/ independent bathing	—tub seat or shower chair —hand-held spray —bath mitt with pocket for soap
	writing	—pencil laced between fingers may be used —built-up writing utensils —felt tipped pens
	typing	—pencil laced between fingers may be used —electric typewriter
	using a telephone	—pencil laced between fingers may be used —touch tone telephone —automatic dial telephone
	cooking	—wheelchair accessible work surfaces —wheelchair accessible appliances —other adaptive kitchen equipment as indicated
	driving a car (with independent car transfer)	—hand controls —steering knob or cuff
	return to school (can be mainstreamed)	—electric typewriter —wheelchair bag for carrying supplies —tape recorder for taking notes —computer

Table II cont.

LEVEL AND FUNCTION REMAINING	TREATMENT GUIDELINES	FUNCTIONAL OBJECTIVE	FUNCTIONAL EQUIPMENT
C_8 to T_4 good to normal upper extremity function	—passive range of motion (teach self-range) *Note*: less than normal range is desirable in the back extensors. Greater than normal range is desirable in the hamstrings.	increase tolerance to upright position	—tilt table—manual or electric —reclining wheelchair with cushion, elevating leg rests and trunkal supports *Note*: see C_6
	—strengthen remaining musculature —increase general endurance and conditioning	relieve ischial pressure	—arms of wheelchair used for sitting pushups —wheelchair cushion
	—establish positioning alternatives (see C_7)		—mirror with or without gooseneck
	—teach compensatory body management skills	independent skin inspection	—bath or shower chair
	—teach pressure relief techniques including wheelchair pushups and use of cushion	independent bathing independent transfers independent community mobility	—sliding board may be used —into wheelchair- accessible buildings —sidewalk ramps —in wheelchair-
	—teach ADLs (see C_7)	independent cooking	—accessible kitchen
	—ambulation training for the younger patient		—in wheelchair- accessible house
	—train for wheelchair mobility in the community	independent light housekeeping (may not be energy efficient)	
	—train in use of adaptive equipment —explore alternatives for prevocational/vocational training	return to school	—manual wheelchair with tray —wheelchair bag for supplies
	—patient and family training in physical care, functional activities, use and maintenance of all equipment		
	—provide home program		

Level	Treatment	Goals	Equipment
T₅ to L₂ partial to good trunk stability increased endurance due to larger respiratory reserve	—passive range of motion (teach self-range) *Note:* greater than normal range is desirable in the hamstrings —strengthen remaining musculature —increase general endurance and conditioning —establish positioning alternatives —teach compensatory body management skills —teach pressure relief techniques including wheelchair pushups and use of cushion —teach ADLs including hygiene, dressing, bathing, skin care, transfers, and homemaking skills —ambulation training (function and endurance will depend on level) —train for community mobility (wheelchair or ambulation) —train in the use of adaptive equipment —explore alternatives for prevocational/vocational training —patient and family training in physical care, functional activities, use and maintenance of all equipment —provide home program	independent self-care wheelchair mobility ambulation (for short distances) independent house-keeping return to school	—bathtub bench or shower chair —mirror for skin inspection —standard or low-backed wheelchair —bilateral long leg braces with or without pelvic band —crutches —in wheelchair-accessible house —manual wheelchair with tray —wheelchair bag for supplies
L³⁻⁴ pelvic-trunk stabilizers hip flexors, adductors, quadriceps	—teach self-range if indicated —strengthen remaining musculature —increase general endurance and conditioning	independent self-care independent ambulation	—no equipment necessary —short leg braces or molded ankle/foot orthosis (MAFOs) —crutches or canes may be used

Table II cont.

LEVEL AND FUNCTION REMAINING	TREATMENT GUIDELINES	FUNCTIONAL OBJECTIVE	FUNCTIONAL EQUIPMENT
L3-4	—teach compensatory body management skills —teach awareness of pressure areas —teach ADLs including hygiene, dressing, bathing, skin care and homemaking skills —ambulation training —train for community mobility —train in the use and maintenance of braces/MAFOs if indicated —explore alternatives for prevocational/vocational training —patient and family training in physical care, functional activities, use and maintenance of all equipment —provide home program	independent housekeeping return to school	—no equipment necessary —backpack for supplies if crutches or canes are used
L5 to S3 hip extensors, abductors knee flexors ankle control	—teach self-range if indicated —strengthen remaining musculature —increase general endurance and conditioning —teach compensatory body management skills —teach awareness of pressure areas	independent self-care independent ambulation independent housekeeping return to school	—no equipment necessary —MAFOs may be used —crutches or canes may be used —no equipment necessary —backpack for supplies if crutches or canes are used

L₅ to S₃

—teach ADLs including hygiene, dressing, bathing, skin care, and homemaking skills
—ambulation training
—train for community mobility
—train in the use and maintenance of braces/MAFOs if indicated
—explore alternatives for prevocational/vocational training
—patient and family training in physical care, functional activities, use and maintenance of all equipment
—provide home program

RECREATION AND LEISURE ACTIVITIES

Recreation and development of age-appropriate leisure time activities are as important for the child and adolescent with spinal cord injury as they are for other children. They provide not only opportunities for physical and cognitive development but also mechanisms for release of excess physical and emotional energy. Involvement in recreational activities may promote feelings of accomplishment and self-worth and help prevent or alleviate depression. Many recreational activities are social in nature and, therefore, facilitate reentry into the social life for family and community.[8]

Often, the patient with a spinal cord injury is able to continue to pursue interests that have been enjoyed prior to injury. For the patient to resume these activities, it may be necessary to either adapt the activity itself or provide adaptive devices for the patient. When adaptations are not possible, it may be necessary to encourage the development of new leisure time interests (Fig. 2).

PSYCHOSOCIAL ISSUES

Health care professionals must bear in mind that the family plays an important and pivotal role in the treatment program of their child. Grandparents and siblings also frequently are involved in the outcome, although the mother usually bears the brunt of the long-term care of small children. The stress of a chronic physical disability in a child often has a significant adverse effect, not only on the patient, but on all family members.[6,26,31,58,59]

The classic reaction of those confronted with a catastrophic diagnosis such as spinal cord injury is well known. Initially, the family and school-age patients experience shock and deny the severity of the trauma. Involved members find it difficult to assimilate medical information given to them during this time. When they are able to acknowledge the reality of their loss they experience grief, frequently accompanied by anger, anxiety, fear, and later, depression. The health care team must appreciate the strength of these often poorly articulated reactions in interpreting behavior. Anger may be generalized and directed toward the health care team. Children may display regressive behavior, negativism, poor compliance, irritability, or aggression. They may become withdrawn, sullen, and noncommunicative, often refusing to eat and may experience periods of protracted crying and inability to sleep. Refusal to eat and other self-destructive behavior may be an indirect expression of suicidal ideation.[7] Even in children suicidal thoughts often occur when their loss and problems are perceived as insurmountable. The emotional status of very young children is best observed through their play. Although Anderson and Schutt reported a plausity of behavioral problems in children with spinal cord injury, this may not be the case.[3] The major tasks of adolescents are to develop a basic self-image, which includes a sexual identity; select a vocational choice; and separate from parents. All three tasks are interrupted by the spinal cord injury. This interruption of normal progress can foster abnormal dependency and lead to infantalization of the adolescent from which he/she may never emerge unless the family and patient are helped to explore other ways of achieving physical and emotional independence.[30,36,51]

Development of treatment programs and objectives is complicated by the fact that the patient may be in one stage of the shock, denial, depression cycle and family members may be in another stage. Each patient's program must be highly individualized as children of the same developmental age with identical disabilities may be affected in a different manner because of the numerous variables in the child's present and previous environmental experiences as well as by genetic and biologic potentials.[38] The best antidote for depression in both the child and family is early

Ages	Patients with Paraplegia	Patients with Quadriplegia
1–3 yrs.	Scootering–use crawligators, scooter boards Blocks, ring stack, other toys–may need equipment such as floorsitters to maintain sitting for floor play Play dough, finger paint, paste, water play–if in wheelchair, may need tray; if splinted for standing, may need standing table Swimming–use vest type floats Swings–may require chair type seat Musical toys	Musical toys–require easy-to-push controls Stack toys–(to be knocked over) Switch-operated toys–require appropriate switch hook up (touch access control) Ball play–use nerf ball, balloon Books–mouthstick or pencil eraser in universal cuff to turn pages, angled surface to hold book Swimming–use vest type floats Dolls–large dolls with velcro closure clothing Water play–need accessible play surface for wheelchair or standing board, appropriate support for floor play
4–6 yrs.	Swimming–vest type float, leg floats Tricycling–hand-propelled tricycle Sledding–may require back support built onto sled Horseback riding–established programs for the handicapped are available Wheelchair sports–nerf balls, large bats, hoop games	Puzzles–large knobs on puzzle pieces Coloring, pasting–may require built-up handles, mouthstick, universal cuff, electric scissors Switch-operated toys, radio, TV–requires appropriate switch hookup (touch access control) Board games, cards–may need large pieces to board games, card holder Books–electric page turner, mouthstick or pencil eraser in universal cuff to turn pages, angled surface to hold book Blowing bubbles, water play–may need universal cuff, tray for wheelchair
7–12 yrs.	Wheelchair sports–baseball, basketball, archery, bowling, pool, pinball, table tennis (lightweight sport model wheelchairs are available)	Switch-operated games, radio, TV–requires appropriate switch hookup (touch access control)

Ages	Patients with Paraplegia	Patients with Quadriplegia
	Crafts, models–need accessible work space (wheelchair or standing) Computer games Board games–need accessible table or wheelchair tray or appropriate support for floor play Musical instruments Scouting–with community group or scouting for the handicapped Fishing Horseback riding–established programs for the handicapped are available	Computer games–may require mouthstick, universal cuff, switch hookup (touch access control) Board games Books–may use talking books with appropriate switch hookup Scouting–scouting for handicapped is available
13–17 yrs.	Wheelchair sports, dancing–baseball, basketball, archery, bowling, pool, pinball, table tennis, weightlifting Wheelchair accessible hiking trails–pneumatic wheelchair tires are appropriate for uneven terrain Driving–require hand controls Gardening–may require lightweight long-handled tools, raised flower beds, wheelchair-accessible work space Fishing–may use wheelchair bag to carry equipment Hunting–may use wheelchair bag to carry equipment Photography Cooking—wheelchair-accessible work surfaces and appliances Scouting–with community group or scouting for the handicapped Horseback riding–established programs for the handicapped are available	Switch-operated radio, TV, pinball–require appropriate switch hookup (touch access control) Computer games–require appropriate switch hookup Board games Painting/artwork–may require built up handles, mouthstick, universal cuff Books–may use talking books with appropriate switch hookup Wheelchair sports (depending on level of injury)–table tennis with cuff for paddle, pinball, etc. Driving (depending on level of injury)–requires hand controls–may need steering knob or cuff—may need special seat belt harness

Figure 2. Leisure time activities for children with paraplegia and quadriplegia.

aggressive rehabilitation and a supportive environment. There is no standard model of treatment that applies to all patients.

With proper understanding and support, the patient and family can acknowledge the consequence of the injury and begin to make realistic goal-directed decisions thereby rebuilding their lives within the boundaries of the child's disability and abilities.[7] The patient and family may remain emotionally vulnerable and fragile.[65] The reaction to the trauma may be rekindled during any subsequent crisis in the life of the patient. Critical developmental stages, particularly the transition from infancy to toddler age, from preschool to school age, the beginning of adolescence, and entrance into adulthood may reactivate the cycle of grief and depression.

SEXUALITY ISSUES

When addressing sexuality issues with children and adolescents with spinal cord injury, two premises about the nature of human sexuality and the nature of children and adolescents with disability should be accepted. First, by its broadest definition, human sexuality is the wide variety of ways in which individuals perceive and experience their bodies. Second, children with a disability share the same curiosity, interest, fear, anxiety, and excitement that nondisabled children experience about the topic of human sexuality. A person's need for sexual expression is not eliminated by disability.[17] The child's age, level of development, and maturity must be taken into consideration in all discussions on this subject. Every effort should be made to help the child to develop a positive self-image of himself as a sexual being. The rehabilitation professional should never lose sight of the child behind the handicap. All children, especially adolescents, need to see human sexuality as being normal and pervasive, and understand that interest in all aspects of it is understandable and desirable.[16,40,41]

Most parents are uncomfortable discussing sexual information with their normal children and are even more reluctant to do so with a disabled child. Therefore, it is the responsibility of the rehabilitation professional to counsel, guide, and support the child and the family in this sensitive area. Children, especially adolescents, need a nonthreatening, nonjudgmental atmosphere in which to gain information, to discuss values, and to sort out their feelings.

In the rehabilitative setting, sexual information is given to children in small groups (coeducational or of the same sex) as well as individually. Groups are composed of children of similar developmental ages and levels of maturity. It is important for all children to have a basic understanding of the changes that normally occur with maturity from childhood through puberty to adulthood, as well as normal human reproduction. This information is presented in a straightforward manner, using anatomically correct terms. Incorrect information and popular myths are dispelled as the group is encouraged to ask questions and volunteer comments. During these discussions, the importance of respect for one's own body and each others body is discussed, as well as each individual's need for privacy.

Adolescents need understanding, support, and time to build confidence in their sexuality. Their normal feelings of helplessness and insecurity about sexual matters are exacerbated by the injury. A major task of adolescence is to develop a sexual identity, therefore, a major impact of spinal cord injury at this time is an interruption of this goal. A female is more fortunate than the male because she has a good chance for normal sexual development and remains fertile. Although she may not be able to experience orgasm, she can view herself, at least psychologically, as a complete woman. The male, however, may view his incontinent penis as an incompetent one. Depending on the level of the lesion and whether it is complete or incomplete, he may or may not be able to achieve an erection. Males are usually infertile because of an inability to achieve successful coitus, loss of ejaculation or retrograde ejaculation into the bladder, lack of temperature regulation of the scrotum, or decreased spermatogenous secondary to chronic infections.[46]

Generally, adolescents with spinal cord injury need to be assured that persons with spinal cord injury can and do participate in sexual activity and that there are effective and satisfying options for them. The patient who desires specific information should be counseled individually as to what options are effective, practical, and realistic to use according to the type and level of lesion. There are several excellent adult resources available that describe in detail the various sexual options.[12,32,45]

COMMUNITY REENTRY AND FOLLOW-UP

Planning for reentry into the community optimally begins at the time of admission to the health care system. The providers of acute care treatment and rehabilitation programs must recognize that most children and adolescents with spinal cord injury return to their families and communities following rehabilitation. A rehabilitation program that addresses the comprehensive needs of the child and family can minimize problems with adjustment in the home, school, and community.

Successful transition into the home and school is affected by the patient's abilities in the following areas: mobility; self-care skills, including feeding and toileting; supplemental communication strategies, such as use of the telephone, typewriter, computer, or tape recorder; and emotional adjustment. Often the major barriers to smooth reentry into the home and community are architectural. These barriers may include steps, doorways that are not wide enough to accommodate a wheelchair, or bathrooms that are inaccessible to wheelchairs with inaccessible tub and shower arrangements. Options are available to increase an individual's independent function within their environment, ranging from minor modifications, such as the installation of ramps, grab bars and shower chairs, to major renovations within the home. Adaptive equipment also may serve to increase independence and may range from simple, long-handed reachers to more complex computer-assisted devices. These are prescribed according to the patient and family needs. Physiatrists, physical and occupational therapists, orthotists, and medical equipment suppliers are good resources for advice on home modifications and adaptive equipment. Architects who specialize in renovations for the handicapped may be consulted for structural modifications.

Periodic medical leave from the rehabilitation center allows for gradual reentry into the home and community. This time can be used by all members of the rehabilitation team, including patient and family, for the transfer of skills learned at the rehabilitation center to the home, the determination of barriers to independent function, the exploration of solutions to these barriers, the renewal of social contacts and activities, and the emotional adjustment to a changed life-style.

Most children and adolescents with spinal cord injury return to the public school system. Although most patients state a strong preference to return to their former school, the presence of architectural barriers and the physical abilities of the patient may dictate the school placement. Return to regular school programs is usually possible for those who are independent (with or without adapted braces) in mobility, toileting, eating, writing, or other school-related activities. For those patients who require more assistance and individual attention, adaptations within the regular classroom or placement in classes for the physically handicapped are common arrangements. Prior to discharge from the rehabilitation center, team members should visit the school, meet with school personnel, and review any special needs. Patient and family involvement in this process assists in the reduction of anxiety regarding the return to school.

Rehabilitation professionals may also assist the family with exploring options for additional financial and emotional support. These may include eligibility for Social Security income; state crippled children funding; sponsorship by a service club, parent groups, or spinal cord injury organizations. Families may also want further information about special resources for the handicapped, such as legal advice, access vans, attendant care, and recreational programs for the handicapped.

The rehabilitative process does not end with discharge from the rehabilitation center. At the time of discharge, a follow-up appointment should be scheduled with a pediatric physiatrist or other rehabilitation team members in approximately six to eight weeks. Most families have had to cope with a multitude of daily problems and a readjustment to a changed life-style and are eager to share their experiences and discuss problems with the team. The follow-up appointment focuses sharply on the patient's overall status and may include a review of general function with suggestions for change; review of bowel and bladder programs; review of general health maintenance; routine genitourinary evaluation, including intermittent IVPs, urinalyses and cultures, and routine blood count. At this time medications can be reviewed, screening can be performed for scoliosis, braces and other equipment can be checked and adjusted for growth, and the home program can be reviewed with suggestions for changes.

Children with spinal cord injury return to their community physicians for routine pediatric care, therefore, subsequent reevaluations are scheduled annually or more frequently if indicated. More frequent reevaluations may be needed for younger children because of their rapid growth. Often the most important aspect of these reevaluations is to provide parents with guidelines that will help them to work with their children and determine what is developmentally appropriate. They need help in managing their child's behavior and in helping their child develop strong coping skills. The family also needs support to develop their own coping skills. Difficulties and frustrations normally experienced during the developmental years may be exaggerated for the individual with a spinal cord injury. The child's physical and mental health should be monitored so that appropriate interventions can be instituted quickly.

REFERENCES

1. Altschuler A, Butz M, Meyer J: Even children can learn to do clean self-catherization. *Am J Nurs* 77:97–101, 1977.
2. Agris J, Spira M: Pressure ulcers: Prevention and Treatment. *Ciba Clin Symp* 31(5):1979.
3. Anderson MJ, Schutt AH: Spinal injury in children. *Mayo Clin Proc* 55:499–504, 1980.
4. Banniza Von Bazan UK, Paeslack V: Scoliotic growth in children with acquired paraplegia. *Paraplegia* 15:65–73, 1977–78.
5. Banta JV: Rehabilitation of pediatric spinal cord injury: The Newington Children's Hospital experience. *Conn Med* 48(1):14–18, 1984.
6. Banus BS: *The Developmental Therapist*. Thorofare, NJ: Charles B. Slack, Inc., 1979, pp 122–162.
7. Breslau N, Weitzman M, Messenger K: Psychological functioning of siblings of disabled children. *Pediatrics* 67(3):344–353, 1981.
8. Buscaglia L: *The Disabled and Their Parents: A Counselling Challenge*. Thorofare, NJ, Charles B. Slack, Inc., 1975, pp 22–71.
9. Campbell J, Bonnett C: Spinal cord injury in children. *Clin Orthop Relat Res* 92:114–123, 1975.
10. Chapman W, Hill M, Shurtleff DB: *Management of the Neurogenic Bowel and Bladder*. Oak Brook, IL: Eterna Press, 1979, pp 46–59.
11. Chrisp M: New treatment for pressure sores. *Nurs Times* 73(8):1202–1205, 1977.
12. Cole TM: Sexuality and the physically handicapped, in Green R (ed): *Human Sexuality: A Health Practitioner's Text*. Baltimore, Williams and Wilkins Co., 146–170, 1975.
13. Cloniger C: *Interdisciplinary Model for Management of a Person with a Spinal Injury*. Downey CA, Professional Staff Association of Rancho los Amigos Hospital, Inc., 1981, pp 52–53, 85–86.
14. Cristofaro RL, Brink JD: Hypercalcemia of immobilization in neurologically injured children: A prospective study. *Orthopedics* 2(5):486–491, 1979.
15. DeVivo MJ, Fine PR, Maetz HM, Stover SL: Prevalence of spinal cord injury. *Arch Neurol* 37:707–708, 1980.
16. Dorner S: Sexual interest and activity in adolescents with spina bifida. *J Child Psychol Psychiatry* 18:229–237, 1977.

17. Duffy Y: . . . *All Things Are Possible.* Ann Arbor, A.J. Garvin & Associates, 1981, pp 47–105.
18. Duttarer J, Edberg E: *Quadriplegia After Spinal Cord Injury.* Downey, CA, The Professional Staff Association of Rancho los Amigos Hospital, Inc., 1972, pp 26–61.
19. *Early Management of the Spinal Cord Injured Patient.* Downey, CA, Professional Staff Association of Rancho los Amigos Hospital, Inc., 1979, pp 32–40.
20. Erickson E: *Childhood and Society.* New York: Norton, 1964, pp 132–140.
21. Erickson RP: Autonomic hyperreflexia: Pathophysiology and medical management. *Arch Phy Med Rehabil* 61:431–440, 1980.
22. Fomon SJ: *Nutritional Disorders of Children,* DHEW publication No. HSA 76-5612. Government Printing Office, 1976.
23. Freed JH, Hahn H, Menter R, Dillon T: The use of three-phase bone scan in the early diagnosis of heterotopic ossification (HO) in the evaluation of didronel therapy. *Paraplegia* 20:208–216, 1982.
24. Freud A: The role of bodily illness in the mental life of children. *Psychoanal Study Child* 7(71):69–81, 1952.
25. Garber SL, Krouskop TA, Carter RE: A system for clinically evaluating wheelchair pressure relief cushions. *Am J Occup Ther* 32(9):565–570, 1978.
26. Geller B, Greydanus DE: Psychological management of acute paraplegia in adolescence. *Pediatrics* 63(4):562–564, 1979.
27. Gruis ML, Innes B: Assessment: Essential to prevent pressure sores. *Am J Nurs* 76(11):1762–1764, 1976.
28. Hardy DA, Melick WF, Gregory JG, Schoenberg HW: Intermittent catheterization in children. *Urology* 5(2):206–208, 1975.
29. Hargrave M: *Nutritional Care of the Physically Disabled.* Minneapolis, Sister Kenny Institute, 1979, pp 32–50.
30. Hayden PW, Davenport SLH, Campbell MM: Adolescents with myelodysplasia: Impact of physical disability on emotional maturation. *Pediatrics* 64:53–59, 1979.
31. Heisler V: *A Handicapped Child in the Family.* New York, Grune & Stratton, Inc., 1972, pp 62–68.
32. Heslinga K, Schellen AMCM, Verkuyl A: *Not Made of Stone.* Springfield, IL, Charles C. Thomas, 1974, pp 1–52.
33. *Interdisciplinary Model for Management Of a Person with a Spinal Injury.* Downey, CA, The Professional Staff Association of Rancho los Amigos Hospital, Inc., 1982, pp 167–202.
34. Jeffs RD, Jonas P, Schillinger JF: Surgical correction of vesicourethral reflux in children with neurogenic bladder. *J Urol* 115:449–451, 1976.
35. Keim HA: Scoliosis. *Ciba Clin Symp* 24(1):1972.
36. Kerr WG, Thompson MA: Acceptance of disability of sudden onset in paraplegia. *Paraplegia* 10:94–102, 1972.
37. Lancourt JE, Dickson JH, Carter E: Paralytic spinal deformity following traumatic spinal cord injury in children and adolescents. *J Bone Jt Surg* 63-a(1):47–53, 1981.

38. Levine MD, Carey WB, Crocker AC, Gross RT (eds): *Developmental-Behavioral Pediatrics.* Philadelphia: W.B. Saunders Co. 1983, pp 562–600.
39. Mayfield JK, Erkkila JC, Winter RB: Spine deformity subsequent to acquired childhood spinal cord injury. *J Bone Jt Surg* 63-A(9):1401–1411, 1981.
40. Mayle P: *Where Did I Come From?* Newark, Lyle Stuart, Inc., 1973, pp 90–95.
41. Mayle P: *What's Happening to Me?* Newark, Lyle Stuart Inc., 1975, pp 162–170.
42. Maynard FM, Imai K: Immobilization hypercalcemia in spinal cord injury. *Arch Phy Med Rehabil* 58:16–24, 1977.
43. Merritt JL, Erickson RP, Opitz JL: Bacteriuria during follow-up in patients with spinal cord injury: II. Efficacy of antimicrobial suppressants. *Arch Phy Med Rehabil* 63:413–415, 1982.
44. Missel J: Suicide risk in the medical rehabilitation setting. *Arch Phys Med Rehabil* 59:371–376, 1978.
45. Mooney TO, Cole TM, Chilgren RA: *Sexual Options for Paraplegics and Quadriplegics.* Boston, Little Brown & Company, 1975, pp 160–175.
46. Myers SJ: The spinal injury patient, in Downey JL, Low NL (eds): *The Child with Disabling Illness.* New York, Raven Press, 1982, pp 229–274.
47. McCollum AT: *The Chronically Ill Child.* New Haven, Yale University Press, 1972, pp 110–115.
48. Nand S, Goldschmidt JW: Hypercalcemia and hyperuricemia in young patients with spinal cord injury (abstract). *Arch Phy Med Rehabil* 57:553, 1976.
49. National Academy of Sciences. *Recommended Dietary Allowances,* ed 9, National Academy of Sciences contract No. NO1-Am-4-2209, 1980.
50. Nelson WE, Behrman RE, Vaughan VC: *Nelson Textbook of Pediatrics,* ed 12. Philadelphia, W.B. Saunders Company, 1983, pp 21–25.
51. Nordan R: The psychological reactions of children with neurological problems. *Child Psychiatry Hum Dev* 6(4):214–223, 1976.
52. Pekarovic E, Robinson A, Zachary RB, Lister J: Indications for manual expression of the neurogenic bladder in children. *Br J Urol* 42:191, 1970.
53. Piaget J, Innhelder B: *The Psychology of the Child.* New York, Basic Books, 1969, pp 36–42.
54. Plunkett MJ, Braren V: Five-year experience with clean intermittent catheterization in children. *Urology* 20(2):128–130, 1982.
55. Report of the Committee on Infectious Diseases. *Red Book,* ed 19. Evanston, IL, American Academy of Pediatrics, 1982, pp 1–10.
56. Rosen JF, Wolin DA, Finberg L: Immobilization hypercalcemia after single limb fractures in children and adolescents. *J Bone Jt Surg* 132:560–564, 1978.
57. Rothman RH, Simeone F: *The Spine.* Philadelphia, W.B. Saunders Co., 1982, p 1119.

58. Siller J: Psychological situation of the disabled with spinal cord injuries. *Rehabilitation Lit* 30(10):523–537, 1961.
59. Solnit AJ, Stark MH: Mourning and the birth of a defective child. *Psychoanal Study Child* 16:523–537, 1961.
60. Souther SG, Carr SD, Vistnes LM: Wheelchair cushions to reduce pressure under long prominences. *Arch Phys Med Rehabil* 55:460–464, 1974.
61. Steinberg FU, Birge SJ, Cooke NE: Hypercalcemia in adolescent tetraplegic patients: Case report and review. *Paraplegia* 16:60–67, 1978–79.
62. Stover SL, Hahn HR, Miller JM III: Disodium etidronate in the prevention of heterotopic ossification following spinal cord injury. *Paraplegia* 14:146–156, 1976.
63. Tori JA, Hill LL: Hypercalcemia in children with spinal cord injury. *Arch Phys Med Rehabil* 59:443–447, 1978.
64. Tori JA, Kewalramani LS: Urolithiasis in children with spinal cord injury. *Paraplegia* 16:357–365, 1978–79.
65. Travis G: *Chronic Illness In Children*. Stanford, CA, Stanford University Press, 1976, pp 481–497.
66. Trombly CA, Scott AD: Spinal cord injury, in Trombly CA, Scott AD (eds): *Occupational Therapy for Physical Dysfunction*. Baltimore, Williams & Wilkins Co., 1977.
67. Venier LJ, Ditunno JF Jr: Heterotopic ossification in the paraplegic patient. *Arch Phys Med Rehabil* 52:475–479, 1971.
68. Wald A: Use of biofeedback in the treatment of fecal incontinence in patients with meylomeningocele. *Pediatrics* 68(1):45–49, 1981.
69. Wilson JA: How to deliver comprehensive rehabilitation using a matrix organization model. *Hosp Top* 62(1):29–32, 1984.
70. Young RR, Delwaide PJ: Drug therapy: Spasticity (First of two parts). *New Eng J Med* 304(1):28–34, 1981.
71. Young RR, Delwaide PJ: Drug therapy: Spasticity (Second of two parts). *New Eng J Med* 304(2):96–99, 1981.

Chapter 10

SPINAL CORD REGENERATION AND TRANSPLANTATION

The subject of spinal cord regeneration and transplantation is a controversial one. Some have argued that regeneration of the spinal cord has been proved beyond a doubt, while others have claimed that such regeneration does not and cannot occur in humans. Similarly, considerable attention currently is being addressed to the viability of spinal cord transplantation as an experimental and clinical tool. Because of the grim prognosis associated with spinal cord injuries and the inability of other forms of treatment to substantially improve neurologic outcome, interest in the areas of regeneration and transplantation have generated a great deal of research in the past 10 to 15 years.

In contrast to intrinsic nerve fibers of the brain and spinal cord, nerve fibers of peripheral nerves regenerate and form functional reconnections after transection. This difference in regenerative growth has been an enigma to neurobiologists since its discovery by Cajal at the end of the nineteenth century.[1] In the spinal cord, nerve fiber outgrowth after injury is usually abortive, and large numbers of nonneuronal cells accumulate at the site of injury, causing mechanical obstruction and compression of any fibers that successfully find their way through the damaged region. The differences between central and peripheral regeneration have most often been attributed to either different reactions of the peripheral and central glia cells or differences in the general growth capabilities of the involved neurons. So far, the role of central glia cells has not been fully clarified, but regeneration studies performed, especially in the last decade, have shown that central nerve fibers can grow and modify their connections even after the embryonic growth period is over. Thus, it is known from many parts of the central nervous system that intact central neurons will grow to occupy neighboring synaptic sites in the course of a few days if these sites are denervated. This postlesional growth of nerve fibers has been termed collateral sprouting or reactive reinnervation. It has been found to occur in many systems and areas of the central nervous system, such as the spinal cord, corticospinal tracts, visual and olfactory tracts, and the hippocampus. It appears safe to say that collateral sprouting is a general property of most, if not all, central nervous connections. One must, however, realize that collateral sprouting is not equivalent to regeneration. The lesioned nerve fibers do not grow back to their original sites. Alien fibers invade and take over the terminal areas of the lesioned fiber. One reason that regeneration is not accomplished in the central nervous system might be that the sprouting nerve fibers block the regenerative growth of the original fibers by capturing the denervated synaptic sites. Although the studies of collateral sprouting or reactive reinnervation so far have not provided direct answers to the failure of central nervous fibers to regenerate, they have clearly demonstrated that even established central pathways can display marked degrees of plasticity. Knowledge of this degree of plasticity has led to studies on spinal cord regeneration and transplantation.

HISTORICAL ASPECTS OF SPINAL CORD REGENERATION AND TRANSPLANTATION

Humans have known from early times that the integrity of the spinal cord is essential for voluntary locomotion, and that a broken neck, if not fatal, can render an individual helpless. The earliest description of human paraplegia and quadriplegia is found in the Edwin Smith Surgical Papyrus. Nearly 4,000 years ago Egyptian physicians recorded remarkably clear accounts of these conditions. Symptoms were accurately described, instructions for examining the patient were given, and a dire prognosis was indicated.[1,9,11]

In the latter half of the nineteenth century, research began and was centered on the question of regeneration of axons in the transected spinal cord. Experiments of Brown Séquard, from 1841 to 1851, were the first combining physiological and histological methods to investigate the phenomenon. Brown Séquard mainly used adult pigeons, cutting the spinal cord just caudal to the wings. One bird, surviving for more than 14 months, gave evidence of having fully recovered motor and sensory functions. Histological examination was said to have revealed nerve fibers traversing the scar at the site of the lesion, but the techniques available at that time to identify them left much to be desired and Brown Séquard's experiments in pigeons were not repeated.[1]

Interest in central nervous system regeneration developed slowly. Two decades later investigators began to explore the phenomenon in mammals. In 1873, Denton declared that he had observed motor function in the hind limbs of puppies only a week after severing the spinal cord. He believed he saw histologically regenerated nerve fibers six months later. Spinal reflex stepping was not understood at the time, and there can be little doubt that he misinterpreted his observation of the animals' movements. In 1894, Strebe described the invasion of nerve fibers into the tissue between the ends of the severed spinal cords but not crossing the lesion site in rabbits. The concept of abortive regeneration of the central nervous system arose mainly from the studies of Ramón y Cajal. He found that nerve fibers in the transected cord of young animals began to regenerate as they did in severed peripheral nerves but noted that the process lasted only about 10 to 14 days after which the new nerve growth stopped and no further regeneration took place.[11]

The early animal experimentation with spinal cord regeneration notwithstanding, in the early 1900s clinicians began to report cases suggestive of structural regeneration or partial restitution of function in humans with spinal cord injury. Stuart and Harte published an account of a 26-year-old woman who, in 1901, had her spinal cord severed at the T10 level by a bullet, which was confirmed by a laminectomy and observation of the two transected ends of the spinal cord. With surgery, the two transected ends were sewn together and the wound was closed. Sixteen months following surgery, it was reported that the patient was voluntarily flexing the toes, flexing and extending the legs, and standing with support. This case was verified by leading neurologists at the time who, unwilling to concede regeneration of the cord, postulated the possibility of a double spinal cord only one of which had been injured at the time of the bullet wound. The patient lived for 24 years and at death had a postmortem examination. A single spinal cord was found that exhibited constricting fibrous scars at the transection site, resembling those of animals who had survived long after the transection of their cords.[1] In 1927 several more reports were circulated of functional restitution in human subjects after surgical treatments of the severed spinal cord.

In the late 1940s and 1950s, Windle and his colleagues verified Ramón y Cajal's observation that regeneration of severed spinal tracts occurs in animals for a short time only. By the use of various pharmacologic agents, such as steroids and pyrogenic drugs, they were able to extend this period of growth for months and, in some instances, years. They also were able to record the conduction of nerve impulses across the site of transection; yet there was little evidence of recovery of posture or locomotion. Consequently, Windle proposed that neurons of the central nervous system are capable of regenerating severed processes and that the growth process is aborted in the absence of drug treatment because the dense scar tissue that develops mechanically prevents the continued outgrowth of the neurites.[11]

Wolman, in 1966, studied 76 cases of traumatic paraplegia in humans and found evidence of well-developed regeneration postmortem in 12 cases, but the origin of most of these nerve fibers were the patients' posterior nerve roots and sympathetic ganglia. He concluded that there was no confirmation from the study of human paraplegia of any significant anatomical regeneration of intrinsic spinal tracts.[9]

Research in the past decade has firmly established the principles of plasticity, selective reinnervation, and collateral sprouting and elucidated their contribution to regeneration. Neuroplasticity refers to the ability of central neurons to grow beyond the normal developmental period (in mammals, shortly after birth) or to reestablish old or develop new connections. It has been known that regeneration of the spinal cord does occur in lower vertebrates. Not only does regeneration occur, but functional connections based on precise topological relationships are reestablished. There is increasing evidence that some central neurons in adult mammals possess considerable potential for regenerative and plastic changes. For example, the hypothalamo-hypophyseal system regenerates rapidly after section of the pituitary stalk. Central adrenergic neurons also regenerate rapidly, but there is little evidence that neuroplasticity in adult higher mammals is adaptive—that is, there is little evidence that the connections that are established are either functional or appropriate.[3,5]

Selective reinnervation refers to studies on lower vertebrates that show that axonal growth in the spinal cord is highly directed and selective. The mechanisms by which such selectivity is achieved are unknown and would have to be identified and mobilized to achieve restoration of function in regenerating nervous tissue. Collateral sprouting refers to the fact that intact fiber terminals lying adjacent to injured and degenerating nerve terminations will sprout preterminal outgrowths and establish abnormal anatomical connections. This process subsequently has proved to be a fundamental principle of the neurobiology of regeneration.

The lack of success of regeneration experiments in producing return of function following injury led to a revival of interest in a field of central nervous research that had been temporarily abandoned—transplantation of central nervous tissue. The growth of different tissues after implantation into the central nervous system has been known for a long time. For example, skin grafts have grown well in brain tissue. By the turn of the century, studies of transplantation of nervous tissue were ongoing but in only a few, and usually not reproducible cases, did the transplants appear to survive. Cajal, in the 1890s, commonly transplanted peripheral nerves and sensory ganglia with the hopes of transferring the regenerative properties of these tissues to the central nervous system. Thompson, another investigator in the 1890s, claimed to have successfully transplanted pieces of mature cat cerebral cortex into the cerebral cortex of adult dogs with maintenance of the viability of the tissue, however, no definite interconnections or communicating fibers could be traced between the transplanted tissue and the host brain. Other studies in the 1960s and 1970s demonstrated the capability of implanting portions of central nervous tissues into the central nervous system, including the spinal cord. The available literature implied that, while survival of such transplants was possible, the ability of the transplant in host tissues to establish structurally accurate and functional connections was highly questionable. The majority of transplantation research since that time has concentrated in this area.[11]

SPINAL CORD REGENERATION RESEARCH

Two significant reactions of the spinal cord to injury, terminal axon sprouting of severed nerve fibers and collateral axon sprouting of intact fibers adjacent to the denervated fields of the damaged ones have been identified. Neither one, in the natural course of events, results in noteworthy functional restitution of spinal cord function. Terminal axon sprouts when blocked perform synapses on inappropriate structures and cease to grow.[8] All elements of the blockade have not been identified, but enough information is available to permit investigation of measures for extending the regeneration and circumventing the naturally occurring abortive process. One approach has been to investigate methods of aiding the progressive growth of axon sprouts into and through the region of injury where scar tissue forms.

Pyrogens and Hormones

Chambers observed a spinal injured dog that had been administered bacterial pyrogens during the investigation of neural centers of temperature regulation. The dog responded to stimulation of its bladder by howling. This fortuitous observation led to experiments on the effect of pyrogens on spinal cord regeneration. The principal pyrogenic agent used was Piromen, a preparation derived from a Pseudomonas species. The main effect of administering pyrogens to animals with spinal cord transection was alteration of the character of the tissues at the severed ends of the cord and in the gap between the severed ends. Glial membrane formation was inhibited. The effect of ACTH was similar to Piromen. Not only could regenerating nerve fibers traversing the transection site be demonstrated histologically, but they could also conduct impulses for short distances. Voluntary restitution of hind limb movements was not attained.[5,9]

The progress of regeneration in the transected spinal cord of mature cats came to a halt after 8 months or more and in 12 to 18 months, the animals that had been treated with Piromen became indistinguishable from untreated spinal cats. A constricting scar of dense collagenous tissue formed at the transection site. Thus, it became evident that if regenerating nerve fibers were to make functional connections it was necessary to find ways of preventing development of such constricting scars.

Millipore Filter Membranes

A method was devised by Campbell and associates in 1957 to protect the region of the spinal cord severence from encroachment by collagenous scar tissue. It consisted of enclosing the severed ends of the cord in a wrapping of porous filter paper material, millipore. Using this technique, investigators achieved considerable success in adult cats. Even though a glial reaction occurred, terminal axon sprouts were oriented longitudinally and many of them grew across the transection site. However, the millipore membrane eventually became calcified which terminated its usefulness.[9]

Enzymes

That various proteolytic enzymes have been used effectively in the treatment of human connective tissue disorders led to consideration of their use to reduce scar tissue in spinal cord injury. In 1952, Freeman began to investigate possible effects of an intrathecally applied solution of trypsin in reducing scar formation after spinal cord hemisection in dogs. He found the treated dogs regained function sooner than the untreated dogs, and that collagenous scars were reduced at the site of injury.[1] Matinian and Andreasian in the Soviet Union have used hyaluronidase, trypsin, and elastase to improve conditions for neural regeneration of the severed spinal cord of six-week-old female rats. Overt signs of functional restitution were reported in a high percentage of the animals on enzyme therapy. The anatomical differences between treated and untreated spinal rats were seen as a reduction in scar formation, improved vascularization, and fewer cavities in the region of the lesion. Matinian reported that after functional regeneration had been attained, it was maintained, and there was no significant constriction of the spinal cord by dense collagenous scar tissue. The successful result of enzyme studies in animals encouraged exploration of possible benefits to be derived from enzyme therapy in human spinal cord injury. Although little was ever published, evaluation of the results with hyaluronidase and with a combination of hyaluronidase and trypsin in human experiments led Matinian to cautiously suggest some hope for its use in human spinal cord injury. Subsequently, it has since been shown that enzyme therapy in human spinal cord injury is of little, if any, benefit.[4]

Other Agents

Irradiation of spinal cord lesions with x-rays to diminish scar formation was used with some success in adult female dogs by Turbs and associates.[11] Fertig, as well as Williams, found that treatment with triiodothyronine had beneficial effects on central nervous system lesions. Among other drugs effectively used experimentally in cord lesions by Williams, concanavlin-A appeared to reduce microcavity formation. The possibility of using other chemotherapeutic agents has not been extensively explored.[1]

Spinal Cord Reconstruction

It would seem that in paraplegic or quadriplegic patients, whose condition has become static, the one best hope may be to learn how to reconstruct the spinal cord. Modern techniques of microsurgery have been used in this regard by various investigators. It is well known that the pathologic

changes that occur in severely injured spinal cords produced by transection, contusion, or compression are similar
if not identical. The damaged spinal cord tissue is eventually removed and replaced either by a single cavity or a
connective tissue scar surrounded by smaller cavities.

Kao observed in both transection and contusion models
that posttraumatic spinal cord cavitation begins as numerous microcysts at a distance of 1 to 2 mm from the end
points of trauma within the noncontused cord. As the microcysts enlarge, coalesce, and rupture, 1 to 2 mm of mor-
phologically unaltered spinal cord tissue between
microcysts and the end point of trauma are completely de-
tached by the microcysts from the remaining viable spinal
cord—a process Kao termed autotomy. Lysosomal autolysis
of the 1 to 2 mm segment of the spinal cord subsequently
occurs. If spinal cord repair by the surgeon was to become a
reality, then a way had to be found to correct for the effects
of autotomy. Kao previously showed that a spinal cord
could be sharply transected using a subpial microsurgical
technique, and autogenous brain slices, segments of nerves,
or ganglia immediately can be placed into the gap and
closely approximated with the spinal cord stumps. Unfortunately, when this was done autotomy of the spinal cord
stumps followed and most of the grafts became isolated
from the spinal cord by cavities. In previous observations,
lysosomal spinal cord autotomy appeared to be a self-
limiting process. This suggested that rather than immediate
grafting in the injured cord, grafting should be delayed
until spinal cord autotomy had become nearly complete,
which is about one week after the initial spinal cord injury.
At the time, the necrotic and cavitated cord tissue could be
removed and autogenous siatic nerve segments grafted into
the viable portions of the spinal cord.[2]

Kao's result from delayed grafting shown that no
further cord autotomy took place and the grafted nerve had
adhered to both cord stumps within one month without
cavitation. The original myelin sheath and axons of the

grafted nerve underwent rapid degeneration. By the end of the second week, both the original myelin sheath and axon had been removed and strands of neurilemma cells were formed. Axons identified within the grafted nerves at more than one month after transplantation thus were derived by ingrowth and, therefore, were regenerated axons. Bridging of the gap by many axons between the spinal cord stumps and grafted nerve at both ends, the undisturbed parallel coarse of axons within the grafted nerves, and the presence of axons myelineated by oligodendroglia in the grafted nerves all favored the conclusion that these regenerated axons were of spinal cord origin.[1]

Kao using this technique went on to demonstrate that spinal cord regeneration was significantly effective as to allow functional restitution of activity in the lower extremities in dogs. However, Kao's experimental studies repeated by numerous investigators were never replicated. Thus, interest in spinal cord reconstruction subsequently waned.[11]

SPINAL CORD TRANSPLANTATION

As clinical studies of spinal cord regeneration failed to substantiate any significant functional neurologic recovery following spinal cord injury, the concept of transplantation into the spinal cord in order to replace the damaged neuronal circuitry began to take hold in the 1980s. Aguayo and his group in Montreal have shown conclusively that peripheral nerve-axonal bridges can be used to provide a stimulus for regenerative neuronal growth as well as providing a conduit to direct such growth in the spinal cord.[11]

It has been known for many years that peripheral nerve segments grafted between the cut ends of the spinal cord become richly innervated, but only since the advent of modern tracing techniques has it been possible to determine the precise origin of the axons that grow into such grafts.

Retrograde neuronal labeling with horseradish peroxidase was used in adult rats in which autologous nerve segments were transplanted into spinal cords transected at the mid-thoracic level. The results revealed that some axons regenerating within the grafts originated from intrinsic neurons of nearby spinal segments above and below the grafts, and other fibers arose from dorsal root ganglia situated as far as seven segments caudal to the level of transection. However, innervation of these thoracic grafts by long descending projections from the brain stem and cerebral cortex was not demonstrated.[6,7]

In another set of experiments, Aguayo demonstrated that with partial section of the spinal cord and axonal bridge transplants into the brachial plexus evidence of axonal growth occurred from neurons that were situated as far as 5 cm caudal and 3.5 cm rostral to the nerve grafts via the transplants. By tracing techniques, it was shown that some of the descending axons that grew along the grafts had arisen from neurons in the red nucleus, the ventral lateral pontine tegmentum, the lateral vestibular nucleus, and also the raphe and reticular substance of the medulla. The reasons for the differences of the localization of neurons contributing to the innervation of these transplanted grafts after lesions of the cervical and thoracic spinal cord is unknown but may be related to axonal branching or to critical distances between the site of those cells and the site of the spinal cord injury.[11]

Aguayo has shown in various experiments where segments of a peripheral nerve had been transplanted into the central nervous system, that it is possible to determine the origin of the axons that regenerate along these grafts, to estimate the length of the growing fibers, and to investigate the potential for regrowth in several different populations of neurons in the neuraxis. Aguayo's experiments support the contention that the success or failure of axonal regeneration can be correlated with a peripheral or central type of environment surrounding the injured axon. In this light, aborted or limited regeneration after central nervous injury can be said not to be due to intrinsic lack of potential for renewed fiber growth in all central neurons.[7,11]

There is so far no indication of a special population of central neurons giving rise to axons that regenerate into these transplants. Labeled neurons have already been found in several different regions of the spinal gray matter and multiple nuclei of the brain stem, visual cortex, central cortex, and subcortical nuclei. The population of neurons labeled in these studies, although heterogeneous in its location, size, and shape is, however, a small part of the population of cells that normally innervate or project axons across the damaged regions of the brain or spinal cord of these animals. Although this disproportion in part may be due to the tracing methods used, it remains to be rigorously proved that the regenerating axons represent a general potential for regeneration by all central nervous cells that interact with components of the peripheral nervous system.

Aguayo's experiments have produced evidence that axons from nerve cells in injured spinal cord and brain stem can elongate for unprecedented distances when the central nervous system glial environment is replaced by that of peripheral nerves.[7] It seems likely that, within certain biologic constraints, regenerating fibers channeled into a favorable conduit will lengthen until they reach an obstruction or connect with appropriate target tissues. It remains to be demonstrated if fibers that regenerate successfully along the peripheral nervous system transplants can make functional connections with cells in the target tissues.

Recent experimental work by Wilberger using a somewhat different model has suggested that axonal bridge transplants can result in functional neurologic recovery. A dog model was used to determine the ability of a transected facial nerve to functionally reinnervate facial musculature utilizing a brain stem-facial nucleus to peripheral facial nerve interposition transplant graft. In these experiments, a segment of autologous saphenous nerve was transplanted into the brain stem in the region of the facial nucleus and connected to the distal segment of an already destroyed facial nerve. In 50 percent of the transplanted animals, electrical evidence of return of function occurred after three to six months. One-third of the animals had return of observable facial muscle activity. At the time of animal sacrifice, the ultrastructural appearance of each transplant graft was similar to that of a regenerating peripheral nerve. Horseradish peroxidase labeling indicated that the majority of the axons supplying the transplant grafts originated within a 5 mm radius of the facial nucleus.[10]

CONCLUSIONS

With the research that has been ongoing in the fields of regeneration and transplantation, the old concepts of the inability of the central nervous system to regenerate have been successfully challenged. Although many obstacles remain to the successful regeneration across damaged neuronal tracts in the spinal cord, continuing investigation is underway; the most promising work is being done in the fields of transplantation. The experimental work involving peripheral and axonal bridge transplantation for the relief of the correction of damaged neuronal circuits is only in its infancy, although reports are quite encouraging as to its potential for use in clinical situations.

REFERENCES

1. Guth L: History of central nervous system regeneration research. *Exp Neurol* 48, No. 3:3, 1975.
2. Kao CC, Chung LW, Bloodworth JMB: Axonal regeneration across transected spinal cords in electron microscopic study of delayed microsurgical nerve grafting. *Exp Neurol* 54:591, 1977.
3. Kerr FWL: Structural and functional evidence of plasticity in the central nervous system. *Exp Neurol* 54:101–120, 1975.

4. Matinian LA, Andreasian P: *Enzyme Therapy in Organic Lesions of the Spinal Cord.* Berkeley, Brain Information Services, University of California. 1976, pp 1–115.
5. Nichols JG (ed): *Regeneration and Repair of the Nervous System.* Berlin, Springer Verlag, 1982, pp 91–105.
6. Puchala E, Windle WF: The possibility of structural and functional restitution after spinal cord injury: A review. *Exp Neurol* 55:1, 1977.
7. Richardson PM, McGuiness UM, Aguayo AJ: Peripheral nerve autographs to the rat spinal cord: Studies with axonal tracing methods. *Brain Res* 237:147–162, 1982.
8. Sunde N, Zimmer J: Transplantation of central nervous tissue. *Acta Neurol Scand* 63:323–335, 1981.
9. The current status of research on growth and regeneration of the central nervous system. *Surg Neurol* 5:157, 1976.
10. Wilberger JE: Brainstem transplantation with functional facial reinnervation. *Surg Forum* 34:520–522, 1983.
11. Wilberger JE: Transplantation of central nervous tissue. *Neurosurg* 13:90–94, 1983.

Chapter 11

CASE REPORTS

CASE REPORT ONE

Atlanto-Occipital Dislocation

A five-year-old girl was struck by an automobile and thrown approximately 40 feet from the site of impact. She was unconscious at the scene of the accident but began to arouse by the time she arrived in the emergency room. Initial examination showed a right hemiparesis and anisocoria with the left pupil two mm larger than the right but both were briskly reactive. An initial cross table lateral cervical spinal film was felt to be normal. A computerized tomographic scan (CT) was immediately obtained to rule out an intracranial mass legion. The CT with and without contrast was entirely normal.

On a more complete neurologic examination following the CT scan, the right arm and leg remained flaccid and areflexic. It appeared that the child responded by withdrawing the left arm and leg to painful stimulation on the right side of her body but not painful stimulation of the left side. Right diaphragm paralysis was suspected by the presence of an immobile right hemithorax. Likewise it was felt that the pupil inequality might represent a Horner's syndrome. This combination of neurologic findings suggested a Brown-Séquard type of injury to the upper cervical spinal cord.

More cervical spinal films were obtained and an abnormal distance between the occiput and atlas was evident suggesting atlanto-occipital dislocation. A CT scan of the upper cervical spine showed no fractures, however, there was an abnormally increased distance between the occipital condyles and the superior articular facets of C1. Additionally, there was displacement of the odontoid process to the left of the midline. These findings suggested a severe ligamentous disruption of the atlanto-occipital articulation.

The child's neck was immediately immobilized in a halo cast. Traction was not applied because of the possibility of increasing the atlanto-occipital separation. Ten days following the injury an occipito-atlanto-axial wiring and iliac crest fusion was performed. Immobilization in a halo cast was maintained for three months (Fig. 1, 2). Dynamic flexion-extension and rotation films taken after removal of the halo showed good healing and no evidence of instability.

Several days following the accident, the child awoke and became alert and oriented. There was no significant change in the hemiparesis. Three weeks following injury she was transferred to a children's rehabilitation facility. One year following injury she was ambulatory with only a very mild residual right hemiparesis that was evident only under stressful conditions. There was no change in the inequality of pupil size, however, on detailed examination there was no evidence of residual sensory abnormality.

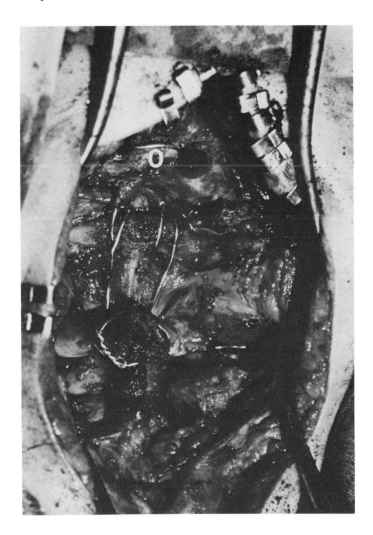

Figure 1. Photograph showing wiring between the occiput (o) C1 and C2.

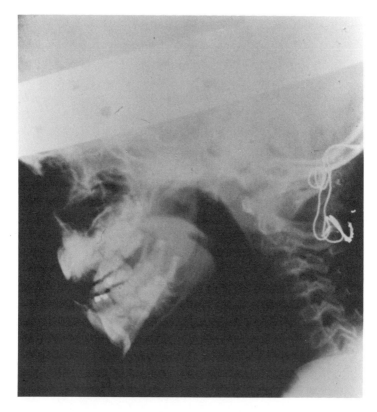

Figure 2. *Postoperative radiograph with the wire in place show-ing a normal atlanto-occipital relationship.*

CASE REPORT TWO

Burning Hands Syndrome—Spinal Cord Contusion

A fourteen-year-old girl fell to the ground striking her head while playing a saxophone in a high school band at a football game. She had a momentary loss of consciousness and on awakening complained of burning numbness and tingling in her hands. She was placed in a Philadelphia collar and transported to the trauma center. On initial examination, she was awake and alert but still complained of severe burning, dysesthesia and paresthesia in both hands. She had considerable diffuse neck pain and marked cervical muscle spasms. Detailed neurologic examination was normal with regard to strength, reflexes, and sensation with the exception of hyperesthesia over both hands in a glovelike fashion. Plain cervical spinal films were normal (Fig. 3).

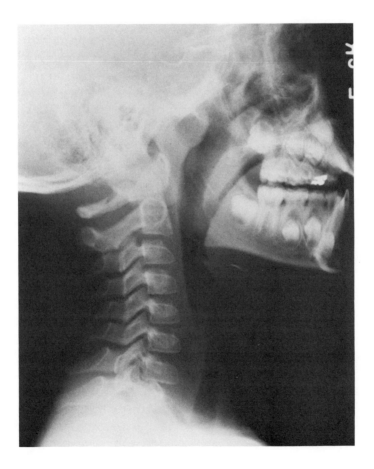

Figure 3. *Lateral radiograph showing no evidence of fracture or dislocation.*

Flexion-extension cervical spinal films were attempted but were unsatisfactory because of associated cervical muscle spasm. A CT scan of the entire cervical spine was normal. Somatosensory evoked potentials with stimulation of the posterior tibial nerves were performed 24 hours following injury and showed diffused decrease in amplitude of all positive waves. A magnetic resonance image scan showed increased signal intensity in the anterior one-half of the spinal cord from C2 to C4, suggesting a focal contusion of the spinal cord (Fig. 4).

Approximately three days following the injury, the sensation of burning hands began to subside. Because of continued cervical spasms, the girl was maintained in a Philadelphia collar for three weeks and then placed in a soft collar. Flexion and extension cervical spinal films done three weeks following injury showed no evidence of abnormality. Repeat somatosensory evoked potentials at six

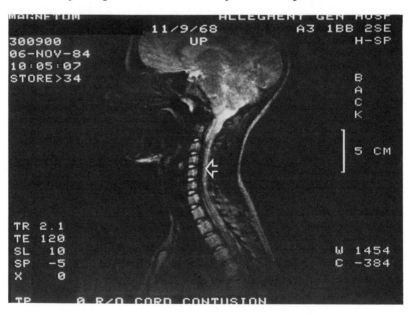

Figure 4. *Magnetic resonance image (0.5 Testa) demonstrating a contusion in the upper cervical cord (arrow).*

weeks following injury were normal. No further symptoms developed in the year following injury.

CASE REPORT THREE

Hangman's Fracture

A twelve-year-old girl was struck by a car while riding her bicycle. She was rendered immediately unresponsive. On arrival at the trauma center she was decerebrate bilaterally with 2 mm equally reactive pupils. No evidence of other significant injuries was present. A CT scan showed a punctate hemorrhage in the internal capsule on the right side and multiple white matter shear injuries in the left hemisphere. Cervical spinal films showed a bipedicle fracture of C2 with a 2 to 3 mm anterior subluxation of C2 on C3 (hangman's fracture) (Fig. 5).

A ventricular catheter was inserted for intracranial pressure monitoring and Gardner-Wells tongs with 10 lb of traction were placed. The C2-3 subluxation reduced without further treatment.

Once the girl was stabilized a CT scan of the cervical spine was obtained. This demonstrated the bipedicle fracture of C2 with additional fractures of the bodies of C2 and C3 evident as well (Fig. 6).

Once intracranial pressure problems had resolved and the ventricular catheter was removed, the child was placed in a halo cast.

Two weeks following the injury, the girl was opening her eyes spontaneously and following commands. There was no extremity weakness evident. She was transferred to a rehabilitation facility where after approximately two months she began verbalizing. The halo was removed after three months. Dynamic flexion and extension views demonstrated good fracture healing without evidence of instability. Approximately one year following injury the girl was independently ambulatory without focal neurologic deficits. She continues to have poor memory and a short attention span.

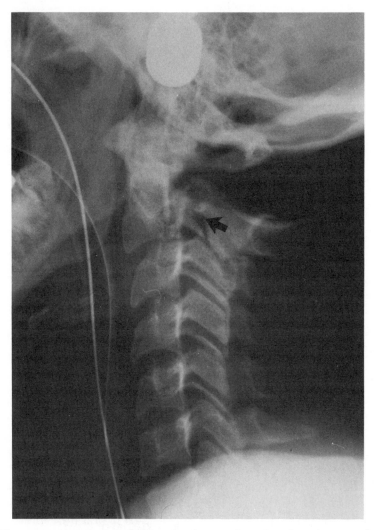

Figure 5. *Lateral radiograph shows the classic picture of a hangman's fracture with bipedicular disruption (arrow) and slight anterior subluxation of C2 and C3.*

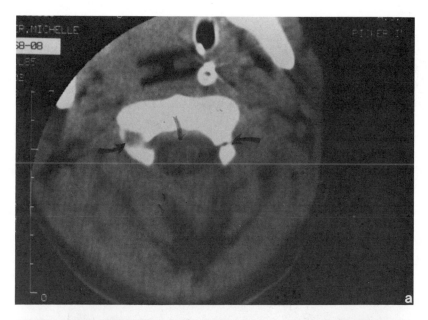

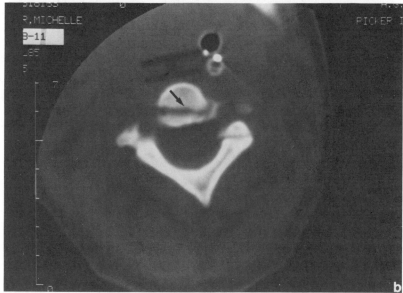

Figure 6. A CT scan through C2 demonstrates fractures through both pedicles (arrows) (a) as well as through the body (arrow) (b).

CASE REPORT FOUR

Odontoid Fracture

A fifteen-year-old male was playing in the family car in the driveway of his home. The car rolled down an embank-

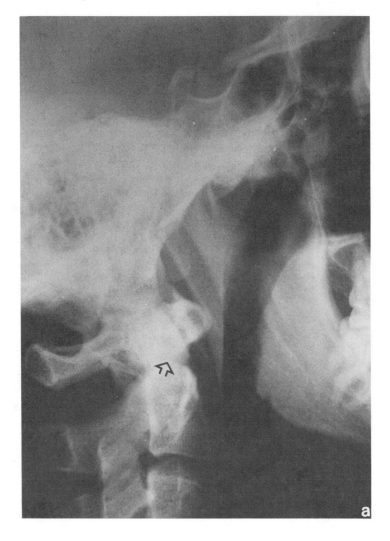

ment and struck a tree. The boy was momentarily unconscious but awakened by the time his parents reached the car
and was complaining of neck pain. He was taken to a local
emergency room where aside from the complaints of neck
pain and findings of some focal tenderness over the C2-3

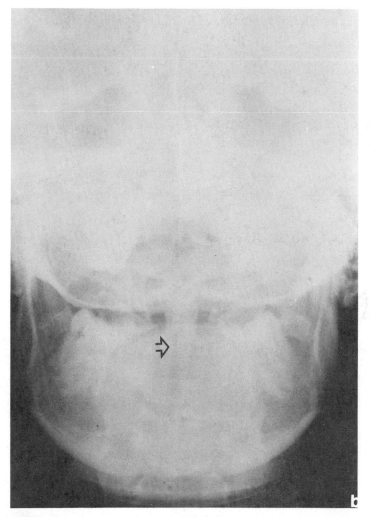

Figure 7. Lateral (a) and AP (b) radiographs showing a type 2
fracture of the dens (arrows). No C1-C2 subluxation is noted.

area posteriorly no specific abnormalities could be found on detailed neurologic examination. The cervical spinal film showed a fracture at the base of the odontoid process with slight posterior displacement of the tip of the odontoid. There was no evidence of C1-2 subluxation (Fig. 7).

The boy's neck was immobilized in a halo cast for three months following the injury. Dynamic flexion-extension views of the upper cervical spine taken on removal of the halo showed evidence of good bony union of the odontoid fracture and no evidence of instability at the C1-2 level. The child was maintained in a Philadelphia collar for several weeks following the removal of the halo to allow strengthening of the cervical musculature. Aside from some intermittent neck discomfort, no significant disability resulted from the injury.

CASE REPORT FIVE

C4-5 Subluxation

A seventeen-year-old black male was the driver of a car involved in a motor vehicle accident. There was no loss of consciousness from the accident. He was taken to the emergency room where intoxication was suspected. A blood alcohol level was 210 mg percent. At that time he complained of some diffuse neck discomfort as well as low back pain. No significant injuries could be documented on examination and, aside from intoxication, his neurologic examination appeared to be normal. Films were taken of the cervical, thoracic and lumbar spine and interpreted as normal. Because of the degree of intoxication, it was decided to admit the patient to the hospital for observation. The patient was kept in a Philadelphia collar that had been in place since the time the patient was transported from the scene of the accident.

Approximately four hours following admission to the hospital, the patient began complaining of numbness and weakness in his left arm and leg. He was also noted to have difficulty with urinary incontinence. Examination at that time revealed an almost flaccid and areflexic left lower extremity. In the left upper extremity he had normal strength in the biceps and deltoid, decreased strength in the triceps and wrist extensors, and no movement in the intrinsic hand musculature. The strength in the right lower extremity was normal. The right upper extremity had normal strength in the biceps, triceps, deltoid, and wrist extensors but decreased strength in intrinsic hand muscles. Sensory examination revealed decreased pen appreciation over the entire right side of the body from the C6 dermatome to the sacrum. This examination was felt to be consistent with a Brown-Séquard type of injury to the cervical spinal cord at the C5-6 level. Additional cervical spinal films were obtained, this time demonstrating a 3 to 4 mm subluxation of C4 on C5 (Fig. 8). The patient was transferred to a trauma center where Gardner-Wells tongs were placed, and with 35 lb of traction, a reduction of the subluxation was accomplished (Fig. 9). The CT scan of the C4-5 level revealed no significant abnormalities except for a fracture of the lamina of C5 on the left side. No abnormalities in the region of the facets could be identified. It was felt that this injury was primarily ligamentous in nature which allowed delayed subluxation of C4 on C5 and subsequent injury to the spinal cord.

Three days following injury the patient was taken to the operating room for a posterior C4-5 interspinous wiring and iliac crest bone fusion. X-ray films taken following the procedure showed good alignment at the C4-5 level (Fig. 10). The patient was placed in a Somi cervicothoracic brace for immobilization. He was transferred to a rehabilitation center approximately two weeks following the injury. At the time of transfer he had increasing strength in his left leg with the proximal musculature almost normal and still no movement in the distal musculature. Left hand intrinsic

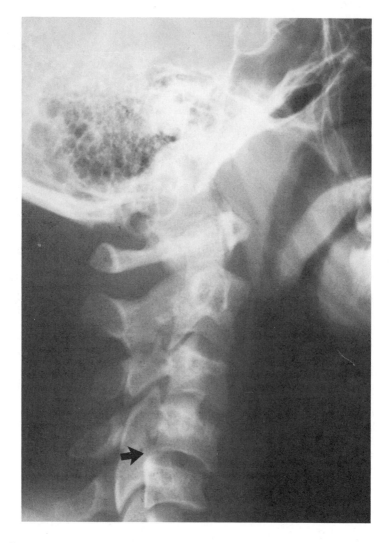

Figure 8. *Lateral radiograph demonstrates a 2 to 3 mm subluxation at C4-5 (arrow). No fractures can be identified.*

hand muscle function had returned slightly. There was no change in the right hand. Three months following the injury, the brace was removed. Flexion and extension x-ray films

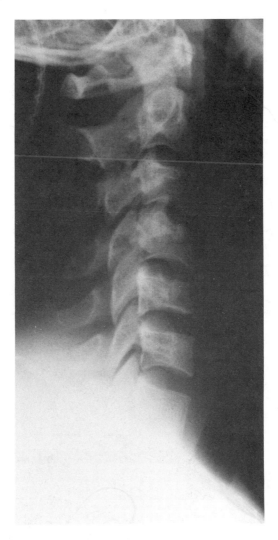

Figure 9. *After placement of Gardner-Wells skeletal traction with 35 lb of weight, the subluxation of C4-5 has been reduced.*

showed no evidence of instability at the site of the fusion. Approximately six months after the injury he was ambulatory with minimal residual weakness in the left foot. He was

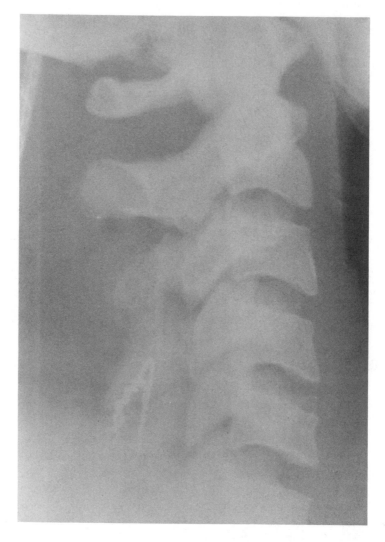

Figure 10. Lateral radiograph showing normal alignment after a C4-5 interspinous wiring and iliac crest fusion.

able to grasp objects with the left hand and had almost normal function in the right hand. There was no resolution in the decreased sensation over the right side of the body.

CASE REPORT SIX

C3-4 Subluxation—Bilateral Facet Dislocation

A fourteen-year-old white male dove head first into three to four feet of water at the shallow end of an inground pool. When he failed to surface, he was dragged out of the water by several friends. He was unconscious initially and gasping for breath, but shortly awoke and began complaining of an inability to move his arms and legs. After his head and neck were immobilized on a backboard, he was transferred by helicopter to a trauma center.

On initial evaluation, he complained of severe neck pain and was quite tender over the midcervical region. His blood pressure was 70 over palpable but with fluid replacement rose to 130 over 70. His neurologic examination demonstrated a flaccid areflexic paralysis of both upper and lower extremities. He had some retained muscle strength in the deltoids bilaterally. Sensory examination showed complete loss of all sensory mobilities including pen, light touch, proprioception, and deep pressure below the C6 level bilaterally. There was no tone in the anal sphincter. Respiratory effort was mildly labored but blood gases were satisfactory—PAO2 96, PACO2 42.

Cervical spinal films showed a 50 percent subluxation at C3-4 and bilaterally locked facets. The facetal locking was further demonstrated by biplane tomography as was a fracture through the superior facet of C4 (Fig. 11).

Gardner-Wells tongs with 40 lb of traction produced complete reduction of the subluxation. As the respiratory status remained stable, three days following injury the child was taken to the operating room and a C3-4 interspinous wiring and iliac crest bone fusion was carried out (Fig. 12). A four-poster cervicothoracic brace was used for neck immobilization postoperatively.

The child's postoperative recovery was complicated by

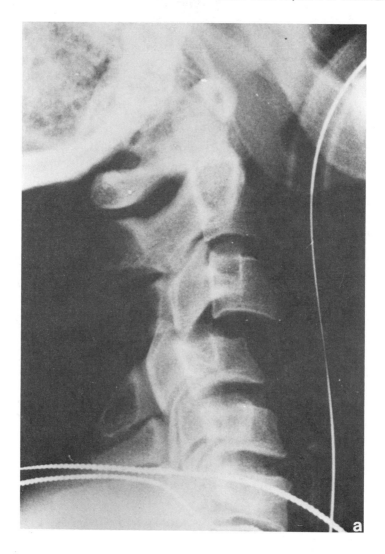

Figure 11. Lateral radiograph showing a 50 percent subluxation of the C3-4 level (a). Biplane tomography demonstrates locking of the superior facet (s) of C4 over the inferior facet (i) C3 (b, opposite).

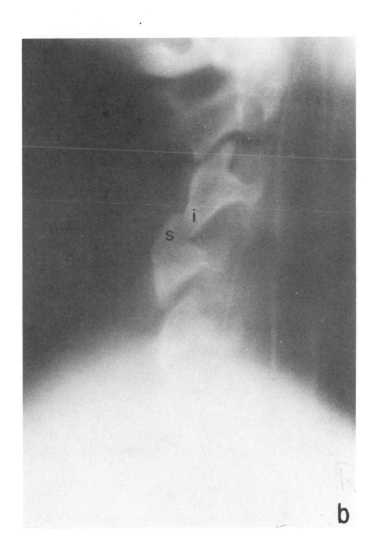

one episode of staph pneumonia, which responded to appropriate antibiotic therapy. The cervicothoracic brace was removed after three months and flexion-extension views of the cervical spine at that time showed no evidence of mobility or instability.

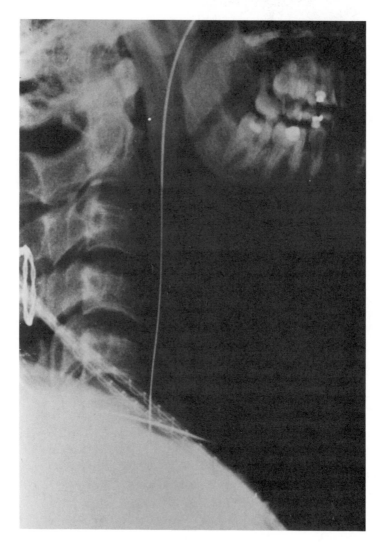

Figure 12. Normal alignment has been restored at C3-4 after an interspinous wiring and iliac crest fusion.

The child was transferred to a rehabilitation center one month following his injury. Examination one year following injury showed normal strength in the deltoids bilaterally, antigravity movement in the biceps bilaterally, and a minimal degree of voluntary muscle contraction in the triceps bilaterally. The hands and lower extremities remained paralyzed. There was a mild degree of spasticity in the lower extremities bilaterally.

CASE REPORT SEVEN

Thoracic Compression Fracture

A thirteen-year-old white female was riding on the back of a golf cart that struck a rough spot on the golf course and overturned. She was trapped underneath the cart for approximately ten minutes. When she was extricated, she was complaining of severe head and back pain as well as an inability to move her legs. She was immobilized on a backboard with her head and neck stabilized by sandbags and transported to a trauma center via helicopter.

On evaluation in the emergency room she was awake and alert and complaining of severe pain in the midportion of her back. She had an angulation of the spine that was visible on examination of her back, an abrasion over the midthoracic region, and marked tenderness and muscle spasm from T5 to L1. There was no neck tenderness or other abnormalities on examination of the cervical spine. There also was no evidence of any significant abdominal injuries. The lower extremities were flaccid and areflexic bilaterally. Careful sensory examination demonstrated that pin prick, light touch, proprioception, and deep pressure sensation were absent from T12 down to and including all sacral dermatomes. The anal sphincter was flaccid. There was no bulbocavernosus reflex elicited. The upper abdominal reflexes were present but lower abdominal reflexes were absent.

X-ray films of the cervical spine were normal. Views of the thoracic spine demonstrated a severe compression burst

fracture of the body of T10 with significant posterior displacement. A CT scan corroborated the extent of the bony
injury and demonstrated almost complete obliteration of the
spinal canal by bony fragments (Fig. 13). A magnetic resonance image scan was consistent with complete cord transection at the T10 level (Fig. 14).

The child was placed on a Roto-rest bed and maintained in a flat position. Two days following the injury a
posterior approach to the thoracic spine was used to perform a fusion. A laminectomy at the T10-11 level was performed and a large dural laceration was repaired. Harrington rods were placed from T8 to L1, and bone from the

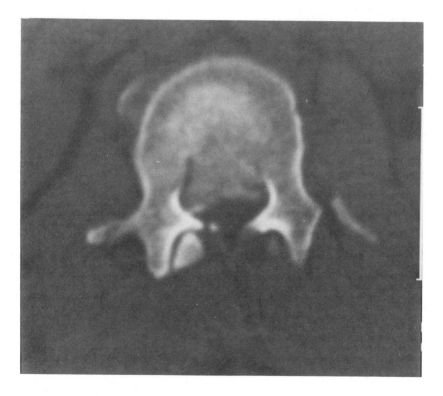

Figure 13. CT scan through T10 demonstrating almost complete
obliteration of the spinal canal by bone fragments.

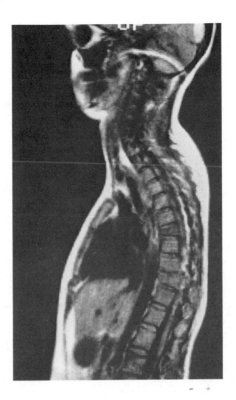

Figure 14. *Magnetic resonance image is consistent with complete spinal cord disruption at the T10 level.*

right iliac crest was laid down over the lateral masses of T8 to L1 (Fig. 15). The child was placed in a molded plastic body jacket following surgery and remained in it for three months.

There were no significant postoperative complications, and the child was transferred to a rehabilitation center two weeks following injury. Approximately one year after injury, the lower extremities remained plegic, however, a significant degree of spasticity had developed. There was no return of bowel or bladder function and intermittent catheterization was required.

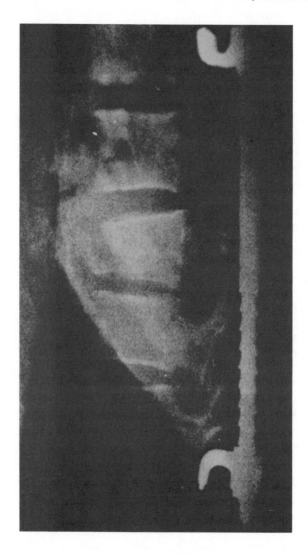

Figure 15. Spine realignment has been accomplished with Harrington rods.

CASE REPORT EIGHT

Lumbar Compression Fracture

A seventeen-year-old white male was helping his father paint the side of their house. He slipped off a platform and fell approximately 15 to 20 feet to the ground. There was no loss of consciousness and he immediately complained of severe back pain with radiation down both legs. He was stabilized on a backboard and transported to the hospital.

On initial evaluation he was still complaining of extremely severe pain in his lower back as well as pain down the right and left legs. He denied any numbness, tingling, or weakness in either of his lower extremities. His examination showed exquisite tenderness over the L1-2 region with severe muscle spasm present bilaterally. In spite of an inability to accurately assess the strength in the lower extremities secondary to the pain the patient was experiencing, it appeared the strength was normal in both legs. Reflexes were normal at the knees and ankles, and the toes were downgoing bilaterally. Sensation was normal to the light touch, pin prick proprioception in both lower extremities, and in all sacral dermatomes.

Plain x-ray films demonstrated a severe compression fracture of the body of L1 with 4 to 5 mm of posterior displacement into the spinal canal (Fig. 16). A CT scan demonstrated a burst type of compression fracture with several bony fragments impinging on the spinal canal (Fig. 17). The most severe impingement was at the L1-2 level with approximately two-thirds of the canal obliterated by bone fragments. The magnetic image scan demonstrated the fracture site to be approximately one level below the ending of the conus medullaris (Fig. 18).

The patient was placed on a Roto-rest bed and nursed in a flat position. Serial neurologic examinations were maintained on an hourly basis, and these remained normal.

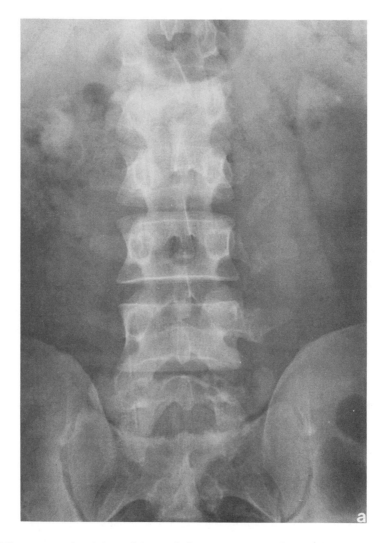

Figure 16. *Ap (a) and lateral (b, opposite) radiographs demon-strate a burst compression fracture of L1.*

His pain was relieved with administration of analgesics. The patient voided spontaneously without the need for catheterization.

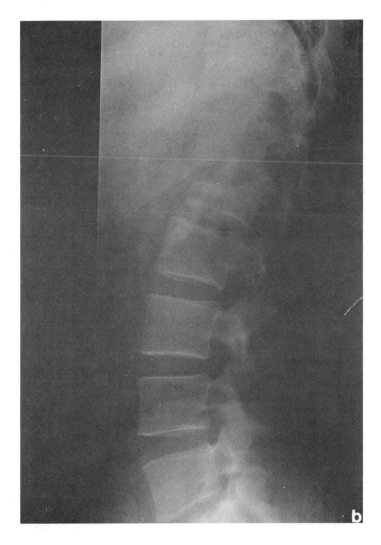

Three days following injury he was taken to the operating room where a posterior approach to the lumbar spine was utilized to accomplish a fusion. A decompressive laminectomy was performed at L1 and L2. No abnormalities of the dura were appreciated. Harrington rods were placed from T10 to L3 and an iliac bone crest graft was placed over

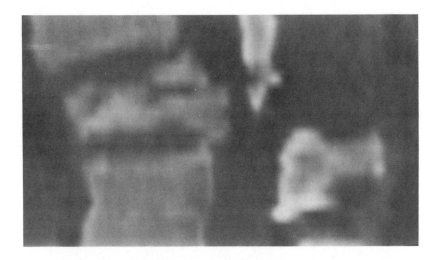

Figure 17. *A reconstructed image from the CT scan at L1 shows approximately two-thirds of the spinal canal obliterated by bone fragments.*

the lateral masses of T10 to L3 (Fig. 19). The patient was placed in a plastic body jacket following the procedure.

By the first postoperative day the patient was up and ambulatory with some moderate back discomfort and no pain in either lower extremity. He was discharged from the hospital approximately two weeks following his injury. His neurologic examination remained normal. He was pain free. The body jacket was kept in place for three months. X-ray films taken at this point showed evidence of good fusion. His neurologic examination remained normal and he was allowed to return to all normal activities.

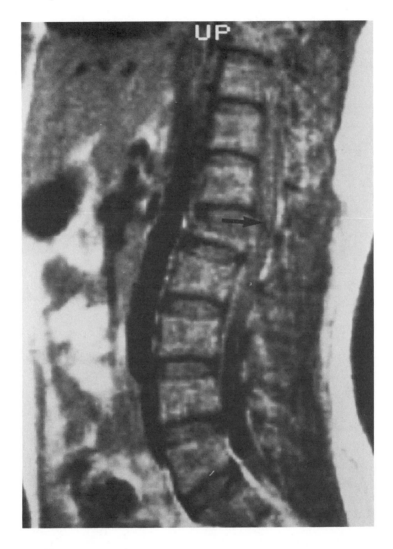

Figure 18. A magnetic resonance image shows the fracture to be just below the termination of the conus medullaris (arrow).

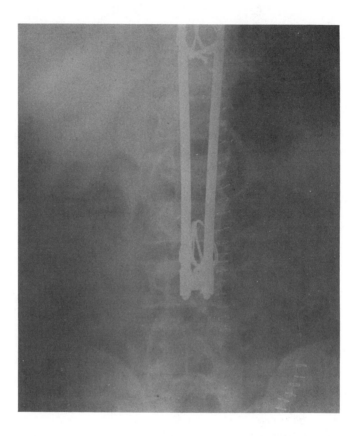

Figure 19. Harrington rod and iliac crest fusion has been performed from T10 to L3 for spine stabilization.

INDEX